The Definitive Mediterranean Soups and Salad Cookbook

Quick and Easy Recipes for Amazingly Tasty and Healthy Meal for Busy People

Lexi Robertson

© **Copyright 2021 - All rights reserved.**

The content contained within this book may not be reproduced, duplicated or transmitted without direct written permission from the author or the publisher.

Under no circumstances will any blame or legal responsibility be held against the publisher, or author, for any damages, reparation, or monetary loss due to the information contained within this book. Either directly or indirectly.

Legal Notice:

This book is copyright protected. This book is only for personal use. You cannot amend, distribute, sell, use, quote or paraphrase any part, or the content within this book, without the consent of the author or publisher.

Disclaimer Notice:

Please note the information contained within this document is for educational and entertainment purposes only. All effort has been executed to present accurate, up to date, and reliable, complete information. No warranties of any kind are declared or implied. Readers acknowledge that the author is not engaging in the rendering of legal, financial, medical or professional advice. The content within this book has been derived from various sources. Please consult a licensed professional before attempting any techniques outlined in this book.

By reading this document, the reader agrees that under no circumstances is the author responsible for any losses, direct or indirect, which are incurred as a result of the use of information contained within this document, including, but not limited to, — errors, omissions, or inaccuracies.

Table of contents

CONFETTI COUSCOUS 6

LEMON ORZO WITH FRESH HERBS 9

ORZO-VEGGIE PILAF 12

BULGUR AND GARBANZO PILAF 15

SPANISH RICE 18

GARBANZO AND PITA NO-BAKE CASSEROLE 21

QUICK SHRIMP FETTUCCINE 24

WHITE PIZZA WITH PROSCIUTTO AND ARUGULA 27

GREEK STYLE SPRING SOUP 30

SHREDDED CHICKEN SOUP 33

MEDITERRANEAN RABBIT SOUP 36

MUSHROOM CREAM SOUP 39

CREAMY SALMON SOUP 41

SEAFOOD SALAD WITH LIME SAUCE 44

ARUGULA WITH RADISH AND TOMATOES 47

SALAD OF COLORFUL PEPPERS WITH BASIL ON THE GRILL 48

SPINACH SALAD WITH PEAR AND AVOCADO 51

CHERRY TOMATO SALAD WITH SHRIMPS 54

GREEN SALAD WITH CHERRY AND PINE NUTS 57

SHOPSKY SALAD 59

SPINACH SALAD 62

SEASONAL SALAD WITH RED BEAN, CURD CHEESE, AND RED ONION 64

GREEN BEAN AND CHERRY SALAD WITH SHALLOT 66

EASY SHRIMP SALAD 68

HEALTHY VEGETABLE SOUP 71

DELICIOUS OKRA CHICKEN STEW 74

GARLIC SQUASH BROCCOLI SOUP 77

CHICKEN RICE SOUP 80

MUSSELS SOUP 83

CREAMY CHICKEN SOUP 85

CHEESY CHICKEN SOUP 88

ITALIAN CHICKEN STEW 91

CREAMY CARROT TOMATO SOUP 94

EASY LEMON CHICKEN SOUP 97

BASIL ZUCCHINI SOUP 99

TOMATO PEPPER SOUP 101

SAUSAGE POTATO SOUP 103

ROASTED TOMATOES SOUP 105

BASIL BROCCOLI SOUP 107

Confetti Couscous

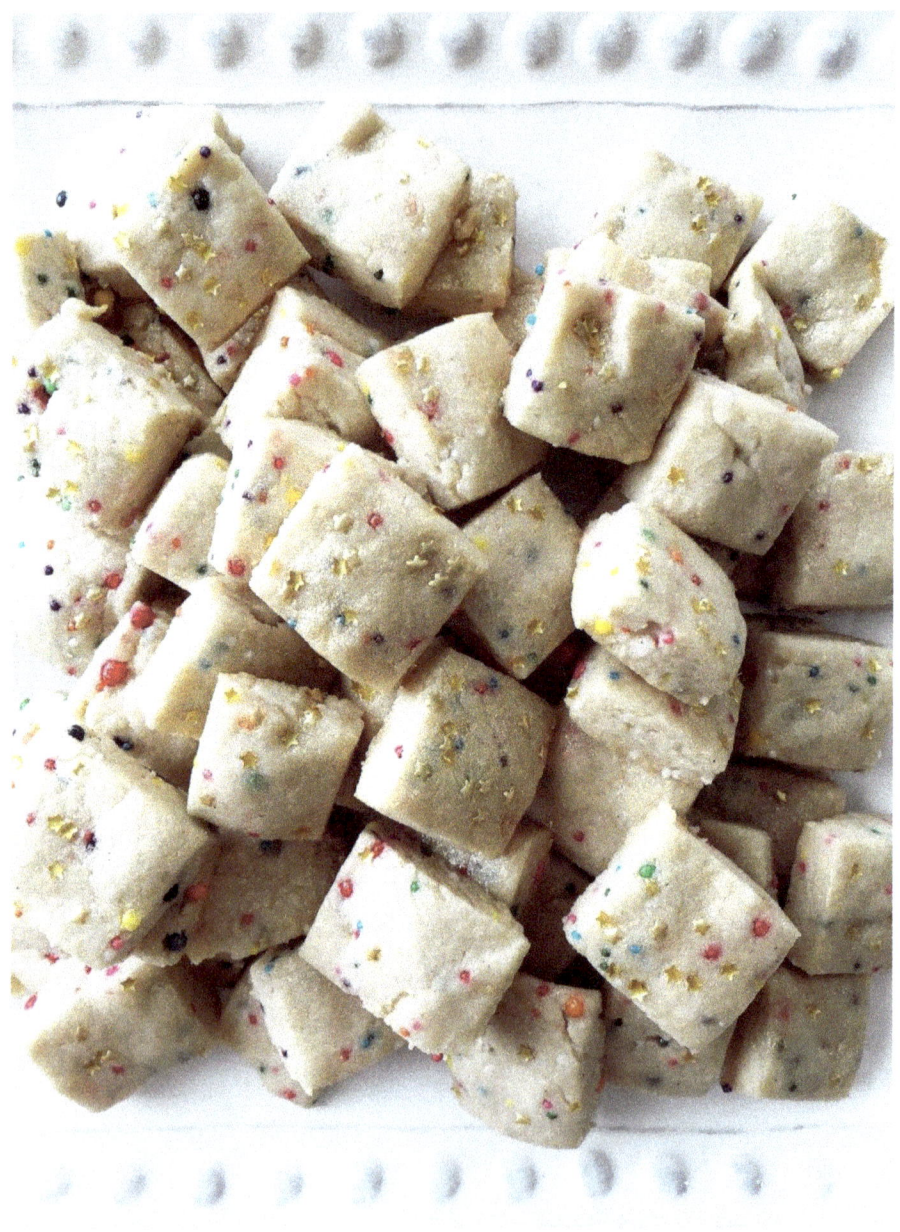

Difficulty Level: 2/5

Preparation time: 5 minutes

Cooking time: 20 minutes

Servings: 4-6

Ingredients:

3 tablespoons extra-virgin olive oil

1 large onion, chopped

»2 carrots, chopped

»1 cup fresh peas

»½ cup golden raisins

1 teaspoon salt

»2 cups vegetable broth

»2 cups couscous

Directions:

In a medium pot over medium heat, gently toss the olive oil, onions, carrots, peas, and raisins together and let cook for 5 minutes.

Add the salt and broth, and stir to combine. Bring to a boil, and let ingredients boil for 5 minutes.

Add the couscous. Stir, turn the heat to low, cover, and let cook for 10 minutes. Fluff with a fork and serve.

Nutrition:

Calories: 511;

Protein: 14g;

Total Carbohydrates: 92g;

Sugars: 17g;

Fiber: 7g;

Total Fat: 12g;

Saturated Fat: 2g;

Cholesterol: 0mg;

Sodium: 504mg

Lemon Orzo with Fresh Herbs

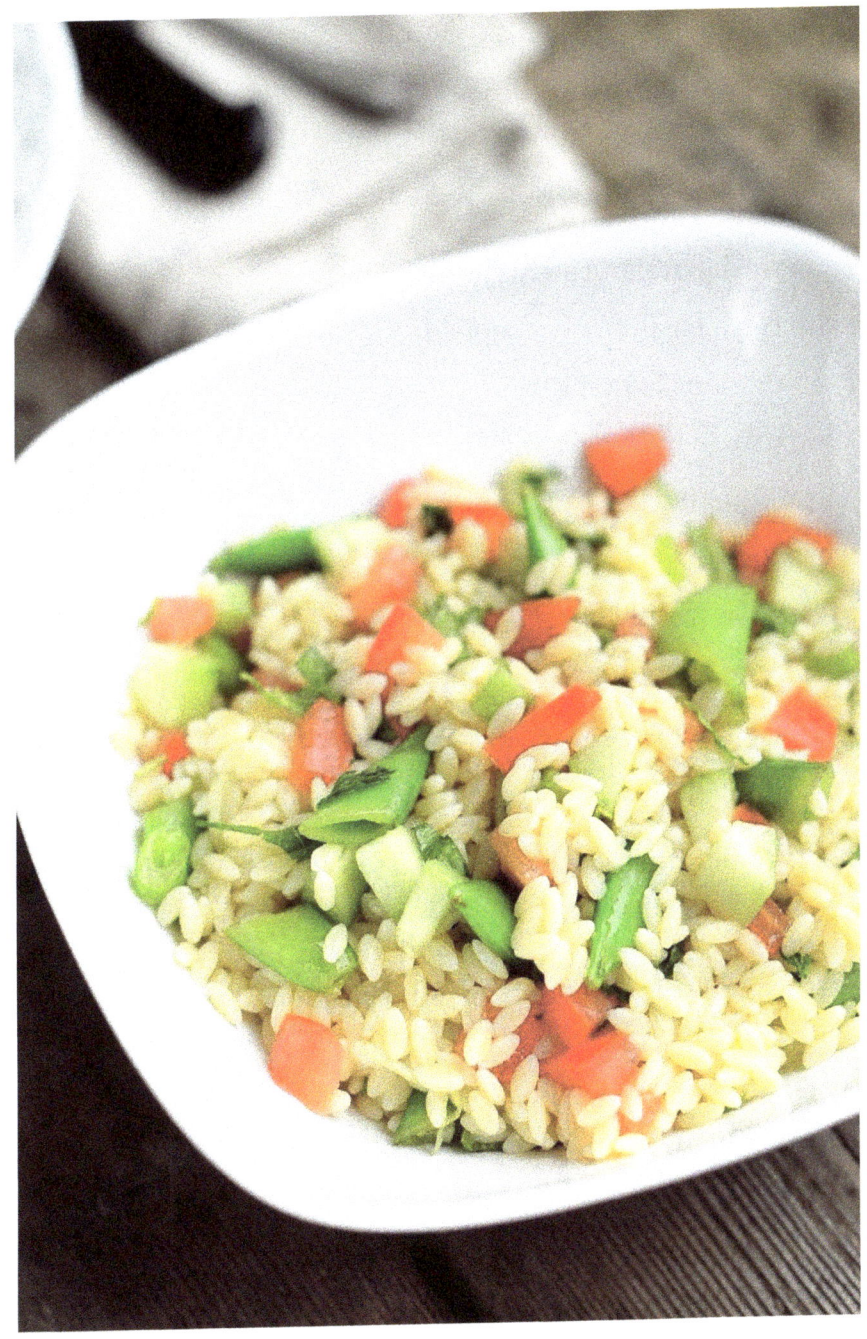

Difficulty Level: 2/5

Preparation time: 10 minutes

Cooking time: 10 minutes

Servings: 4

Ingredients:

» 2 cups orzo

½ cup fresh parsley, finely chopped

½ cup fresh basil, finely chopped

» 2 tablespoons lemon zest

½ cup extra-virgin olive oil

⅓ cup lemon juice

1 teaspoon salt

½ teaspoon freshly ground black pepper

Directions:

Bring a large pot of water to a boil. Add the orzo and cook for 7 minutes. Drain and rinse with cold water. Let the orzo sit in a strainer to drain and cool completely.

Once the orzo has cooled, put it in a large bowl and add the parsley, basil, and lemon zest.

In a small bowl, whisk together the olive oil, lemon juice, salt, and pepper. Add the dressing to the pasta and toss everything together. Serve at room temperature or chilled.

Nutrition:

Calories: 568;

Protein: 11g;

Total Carbohydrates: 65g;

Sugars: 4g;

Fiber: 4g;

Total Fat: 29g;

Saturated Fat: 4g;

Cholesterol: 0mg;

Sodium: 586mg

Orzo-Veggie Pilaf

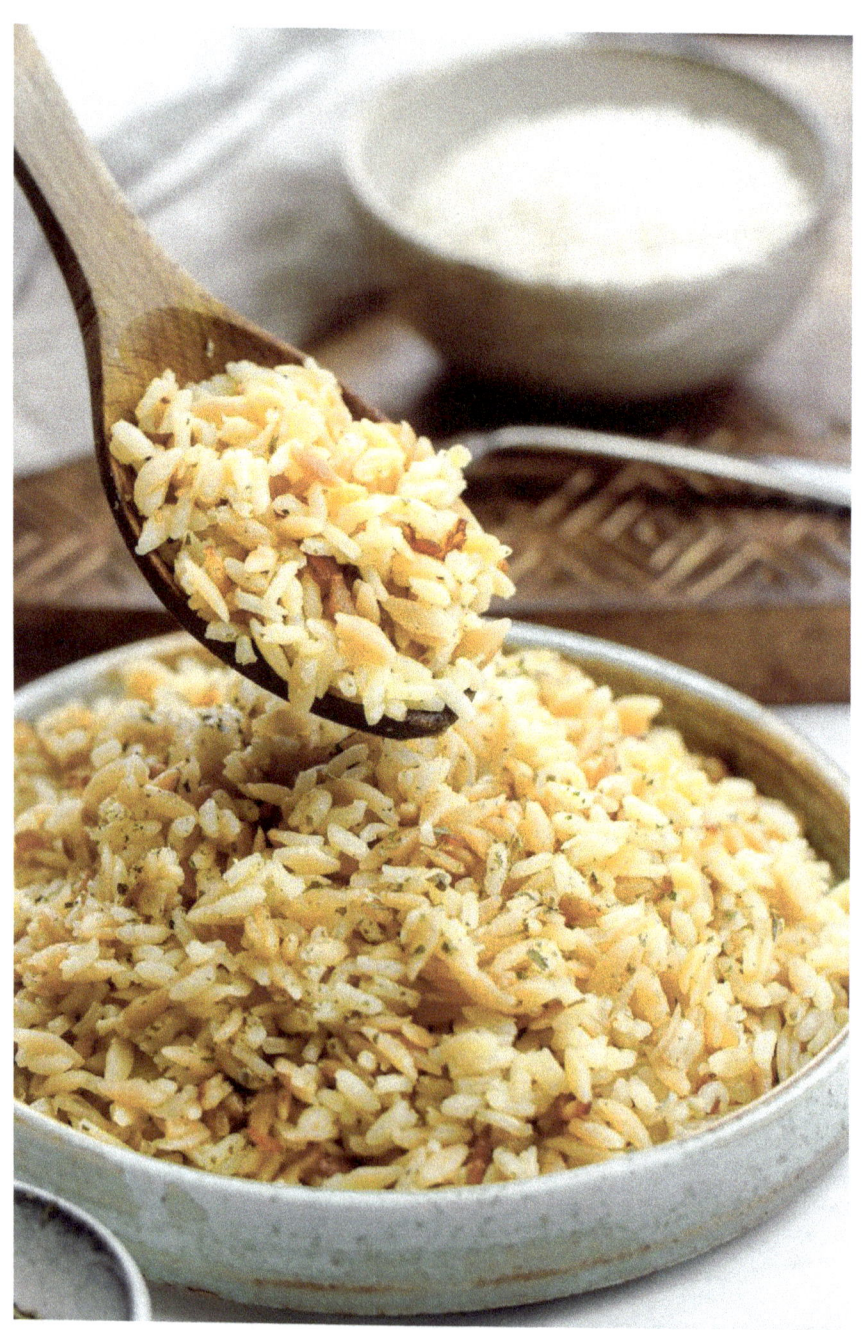

Difficulty Level: 2/5

Preparation time: 20 minutes

Cooking time: 10 minutes

Servings: 6

Ingredients:

»2 cups orzo

»1 pint (2 cups) cherry tomatoes, cut in half

»1 cup Kalamata olives

½ cup fresh basil, finely chopped

½ cup extra-virgin olive oil

»⅓ cup balsamic vinegar

1 teaspoon salt

½ teaspoon freshly ground black pepper

Directions:

Bring a large pot of water to a boil. Add the orzo and cook for 7 minutes. Drain and rinse the orzo with cold water in a strainer.

Once the orzo has cooled, put it in a large bowl. Add the tomatoes, olives, and basil.

In a small bowl, whisk together the olive oil, vinegar, salt, and pepper. Add this dressing to the pasta and toss everything together. Serve at room temperature or chilled.

Nutrition:

Calories: 476;

Protein: 8g;

Total Carbohydrates: 48g;

Sugars: 3g;

Fiber: 3g;

Total Fat: 28g;

Saturated Fat: 4g;

Cholesterol: 0mg;

Sodium: 851mg

Bulgur and Garbanzo Pilaf

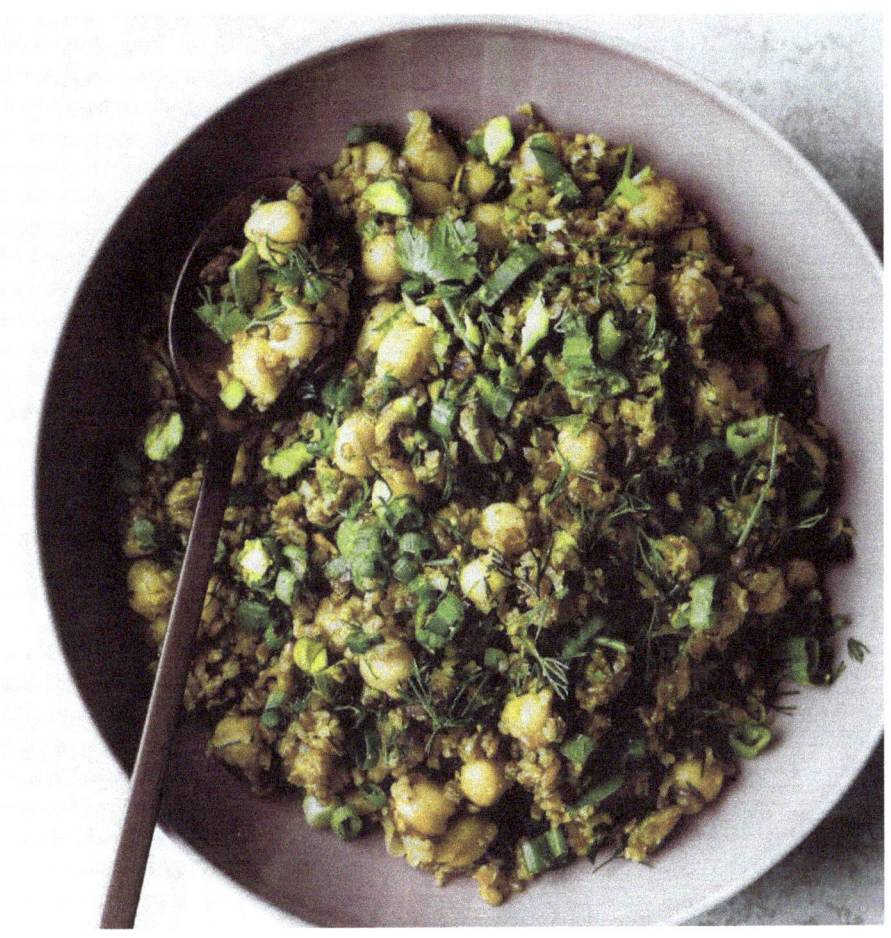

Difficulty Level: 2/5

Preparation time: 5 minutes

Cooking time: 20 minutes

Servings: 4-6

Ingredients:

3 tablespoons extra-virgin olive oil

1 large onion, chopped

»1 (16-ounce) can garbanzo beans, rinsed and drained

»2 cups bulgur wheat #3, rinsed and drained

1½ teaspoons salt

»½ teaspoon cinnamon

4 cups water

Directions:

In a large pot over medium heat, cook the olive oil and onion for 5 minutes.

Add the garbanzo beans and cook for another 5 minutes.

Add the bulgur, salt, cinnamon, and water and stir to combine. Cover the pot, turn the heat to low, and cook for 10 minutes.

When the cooking is done, fluff the pilaf with a fork. Cover and let sit for another 5 minutes.

Nutrition:

Calories: 462;

Protein: 15g;

Total Carbohydrates: 76g;

Sugars: 5g;

Fiber: 19g;

Total Fat: 13g;

Saturated Fat: 2g;

Cholesterol: 0mg;

Sodium: 890mg

Spanish Rice

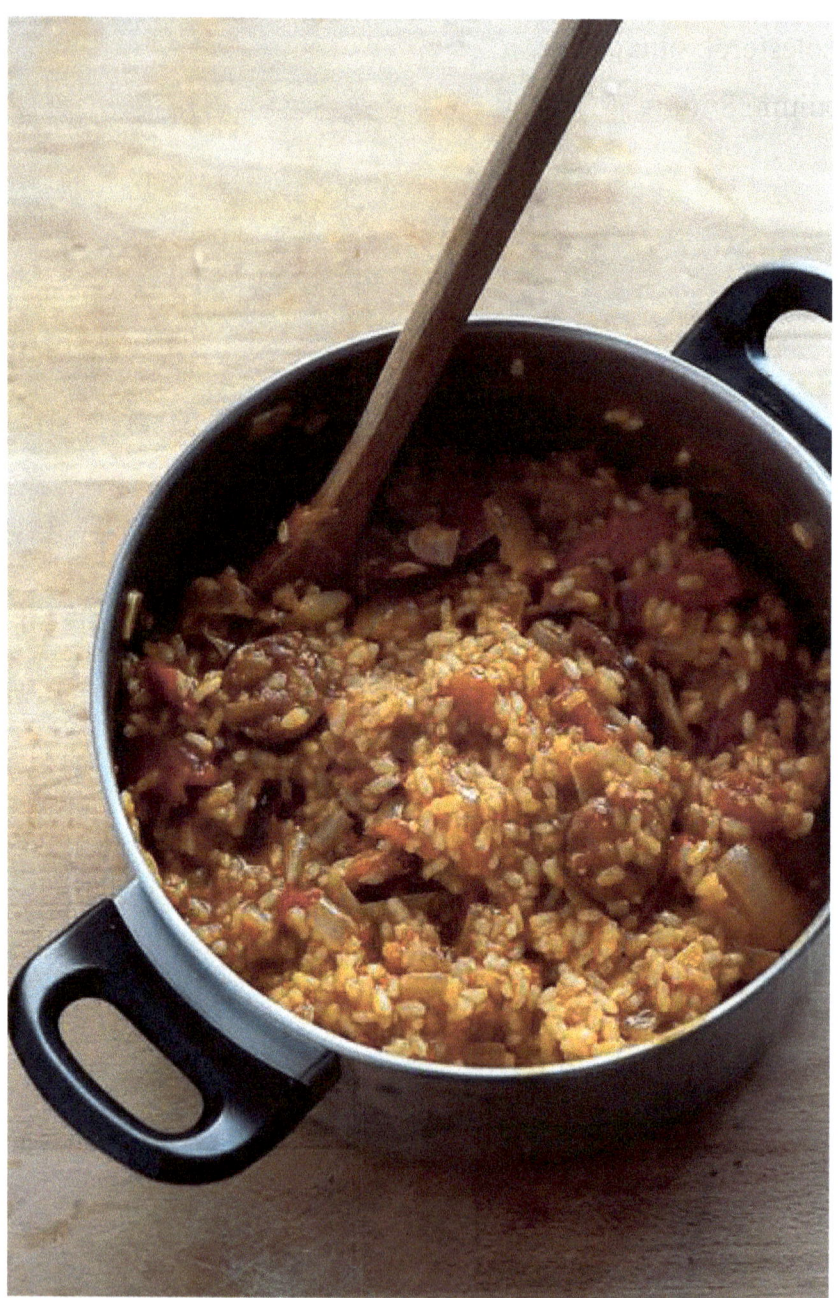

Difficulty Level: 2/5

Preparation time: 10 minutes

Cooking time: 20 minutes

Servings: 4

Ingredients:

2 tablespoons extra-virgin olive oil

1 medium onion, finely chopped

»1 large tomato, finely diced

»2 tablespoons tomato paste

»1 teaspoon smoked paprika

1 teaspoon salt

»1½ cups basmati rice

3 cups water

Directions:

In a medium pot over medium heat, cook the olive oil, onion, and tomato for 3 minutes.

Stir in the tomato paste, paprika, salt, and rice. Cook for 1 minute.

Add the water, cover the pot, and turn the heat to low. Cook for 12 minutes.

Gently toss the rice, cover, and cook for another 3 minutes.

Nutrition:

Calories: 328;

Protein: 6g;

Total Carbohydrates: 60g;

Sugars: 3g;

Fiber: 2g;

Total Fat: 7g;

Saturated Fat: 1g;

Cholesterol: 0mg;

Sodium: 651mg

Garbanzo and Pita No-Bake Casserole

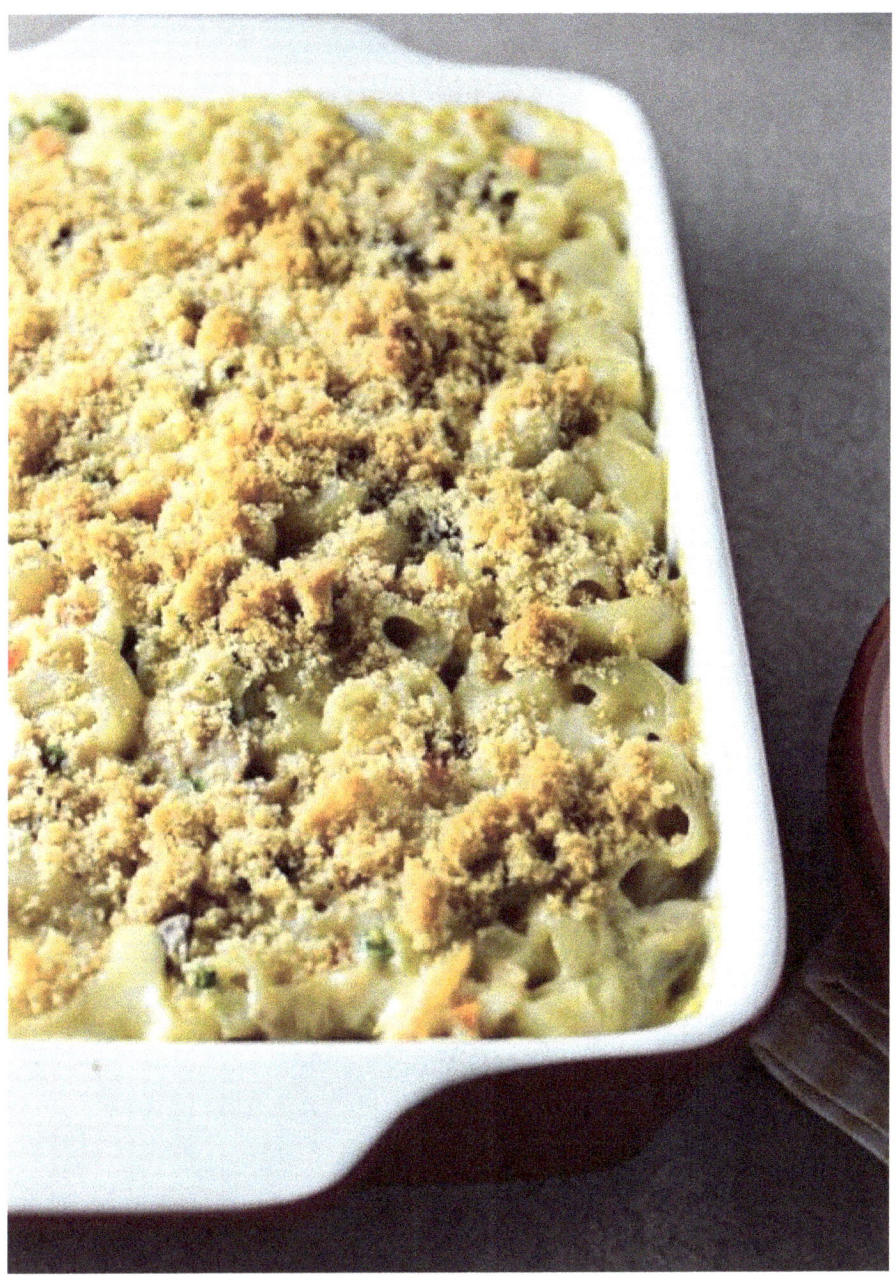

Difficulty Level: 2/5

Preparation time: 10 minutes

Cooking time: 10 minutes

Servings: 4

Ingredients:

»4 cups Greek yogurt

3 cloves garlic, minced

1 teaspoon salt

»2 (16-ounce) cans garbanzo beans, rinsed and drained

2 cups water

»4 cups pita chips

»5 tablespoons unsalted butter

Directions:

In a large bowl, whisk together the yogurt, garlic, and salt. Set aside.

Put the garbanzo beans and water in a medium pot. Bring to a boil; let beans boil for about 5 minutes.

Pour the garbanzo beans and the liquid into a large casserole dish.

Top the beans with pita chips. Pour the yogurt sauce over the pita chip layer.

In a small saucepan, melt and brown the butter, about 3 minutes. Pour the brown butter over the yogurt sauce.

Nutrition:

Calories: 772;

Protein: 39g;

Total Carbohydrates: 73g;

Sugars: 18g;

Fiber: 13g;

Total Fat: 36g;

Saturated Fat: 15g;

Cholesterol: 71mg;

Sodium: 1,003mg

Quick Shrimp Fettuccine

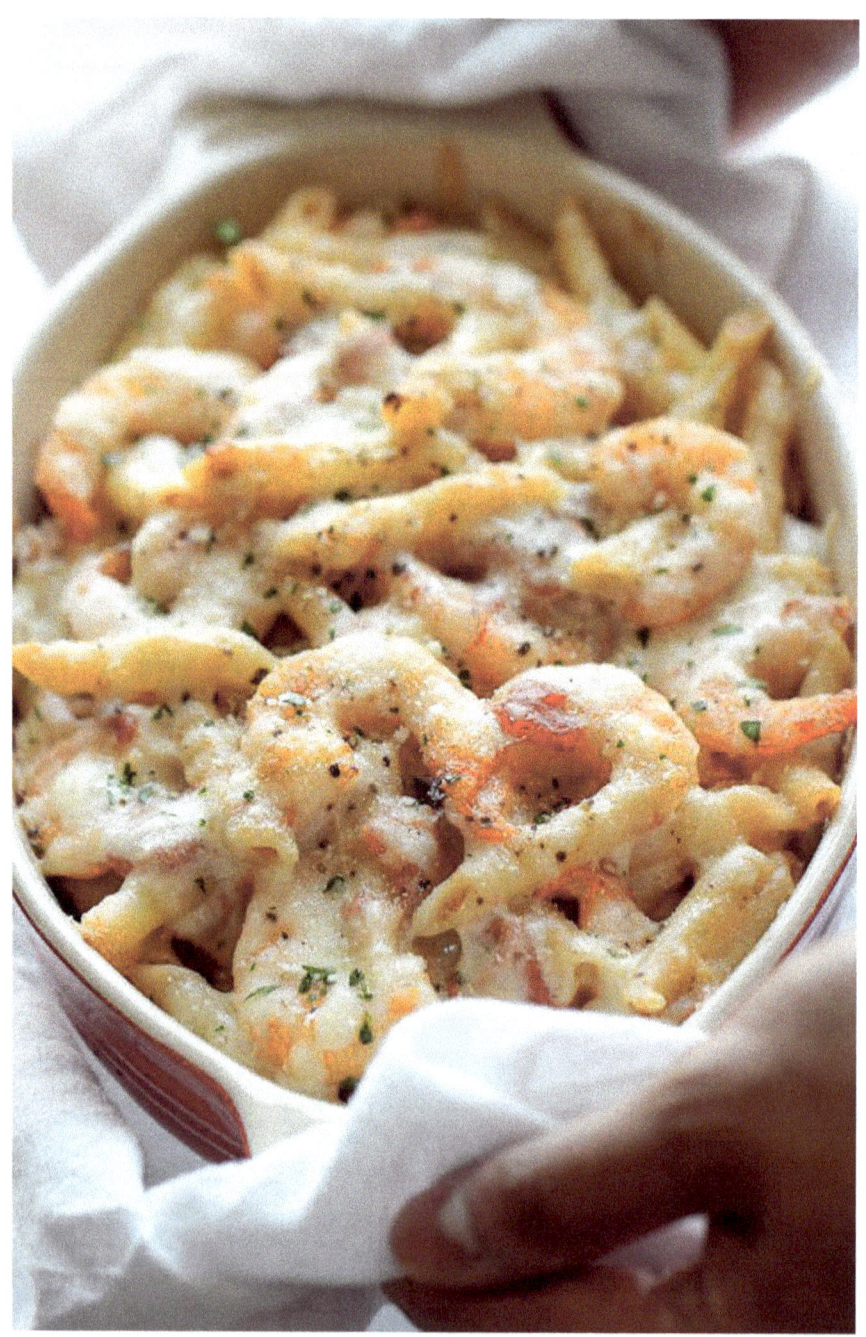

Difficulty Level: 2/5

Preparation time: 10 minutes

Cooking time: 10 minutes

Servings: 4-6

Ingredients:

»8 ounces fettuccine pasta

¼ cup extra-virgin olive oil

3 tablespoons garlic, minced

»1 pound large shrimp (21-25), peeled and deveined

⅓ cup lemon juice

»1 tablespoon lemon zest

½ teaspoon salt

½ teaspoon freshly ground black pepper

Directions:

Bring a large pot of salted water to a boil. Add the fettuccine and cook for 8 minutes.

In a large saucepan over medium heat, cook the olive oil and garlic for 1 minute.

Add the shrimp to the saucepan and cook for 3 minutes on each side. Remove the shrimp from the pan and set aside.

Add the lemon juice and lemon zest to the saucepan, along with the salt and pepper.

Reserve ½ cup of the pasta water and drain the pasta.

Add the pasta water to the saucepan with the lemon juice and zest and stir everything together. Add the pasta and toss together to coat the pasta evenly. Transfer the pasta to a serving dish and top with the cooked shrimp. Serve warm.

Nutrition:

Calories: 615;

Protein: 33g;

Total Carbohydrates: 89g;

Sugars: 3g;

Fiber: 4g;

Total Fat: 17g;

Saturated Fat: 2g;

Cholesterol: 145mg;

Sodium: 407mg

White Pizza with Prosciutto and Arugula

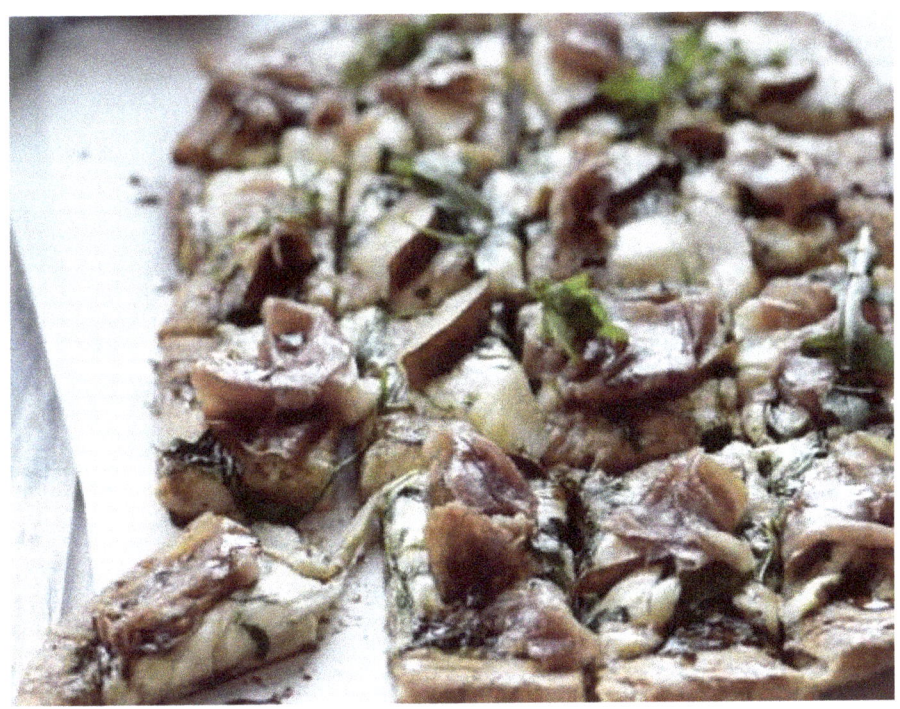

Difficulty Level: 2/5

Preparation time: 10 minutes

Cooking time: 15 minutes

Servings: 4

Ingredients:

» 1 pound prepared pizza dough

» ½ cup ricotta cheese

1 tablespoon garlic, minced

» 1 cup grated mozzarella cheese

» 3 ounces prosciutto, thinly sliced

½ cup fresh arugula

½ teaspoon freshly ground black pepper

Directions:

Preheat the oven to 450°F. Roll out the pizza dough on a floured surface.

Put the pizza dough on a parchment-lined baking sheet or pizza sheet. Put the dough in the oven and bake for 8 minutes.

In a small bowl, mix together the ricotta, garlic, and mozzarella.

Remove the pizza dough from the oven and spread the cheese mixture over the top. Bake for another 5 to 6 minutes.

Top the pizza with prosciutto, arugula, and pepper; serve warm.

Nutrition:

Calories: 435;

Protein: 20g;

Total Carbohydrates: 51g;

Sugars: 0g;

Fiber: 4g;

Total Fat: 17g;

Saturated Fat: 8g;

Cholesterol: 53mg;

Sodium: 1,630mg

Greek Style Spring Soup

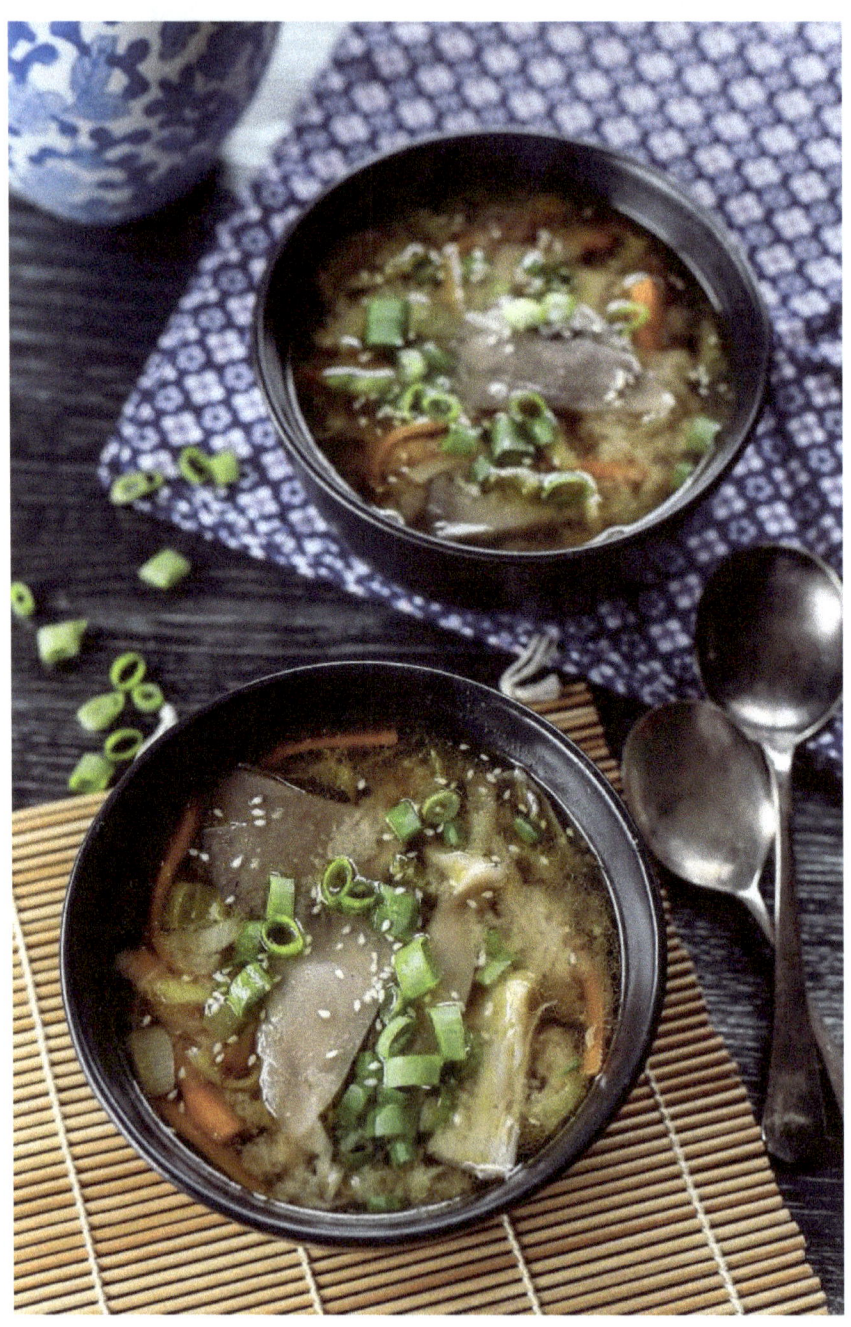

Difficulty Level: 2/5

Preparation Time: *10 minutes*

Cooking time: **20 minutes**

Servings: **4**

Ingredients:

3 cups chicken stock

½ pound chicken breast, shredded

1 tablespoon chives, chopped

1 egg, whisked

½ white onion, diced

1 bell pepper, chopped

1 tablespoon olive oil

¼ cup arborio rice

½ teaspoon salt

1 tablespoon fresh cilantro, chopped

Directions:

Pour olive oil in the stock pan and preheat it.

Add onion and bell pepper. Roast the vegetables for 3-4 minutes. Stir them from time to time.

After this, add rice and stir well.

Cook the ingredients for 3 minutes over the medium heat.

Then add chicken stock and stir the soup well.

Add salt and bring the soup to boil.

Add shredded chicken breast, cilantro, and chives. Add egg and stir it carefully.

Close the lid and simmer the soup for 5 minutes over the medium heat.

Remove the cooked soup from the heat.

Nutrition:

Calories 176

Fat 5.6 g

Fiber 7.6g

Carbs 23.6 g

Protein 4.6 g

Shredded Chicken Soup

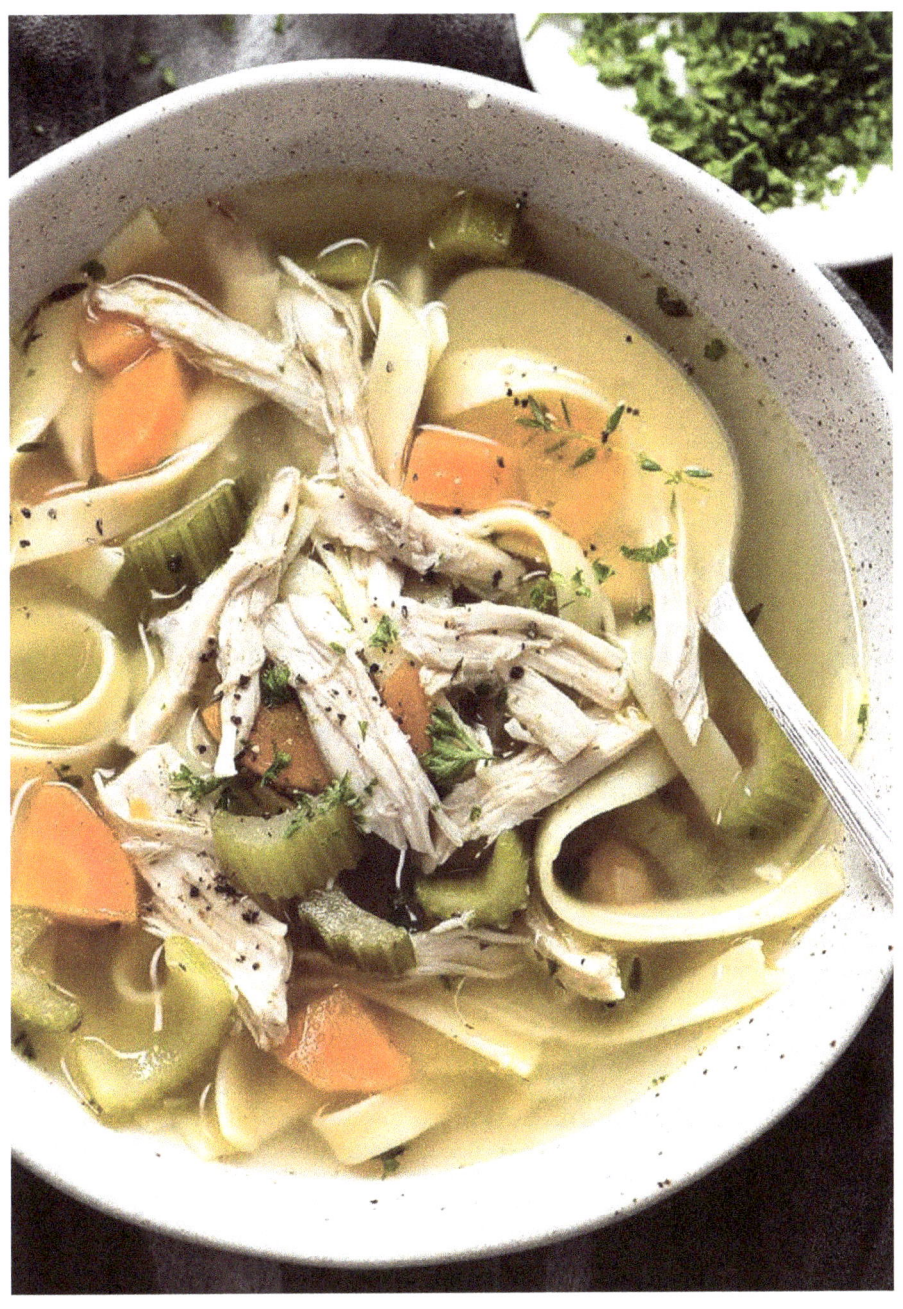

Difficulty Level: 2/5

Preparation Time: *10 minutes*

Cooking time: 15 minutes

Servings: 4

Ingredients:

3 cups chicken stock

1-pound chicken breast, shredded

½ teaspoon dried mint

½ cup Greek yogurt

½ onion, diced

1 tablespoon butter

½ teaspoon salt

½ teaspoon ground black pepper

1 tablespoon fresh dill, chopped

Directions:

Pour chicken stock in the saucepan and bring it to boil.

Add shredded chicken, dried mint, salt, and ground black pepper.

Simmer the liquid for 5 minutes over the low heat.

Meanwhile, toss the butter in the skillet and melt it.

Add onion and roast it until it is light brown.

Add the cooked onion in the soup.

Then add yogurt and stir it well.

Bring the soup to boil, add dill, and remove from the heat.

The soup is cooked.

Nutrition:

Calories 198

Fat 5.6 g

Fiber 7.6g

Carbs 23.6 g

Protein 4.6 g

Mediterranean Rabbit Soup

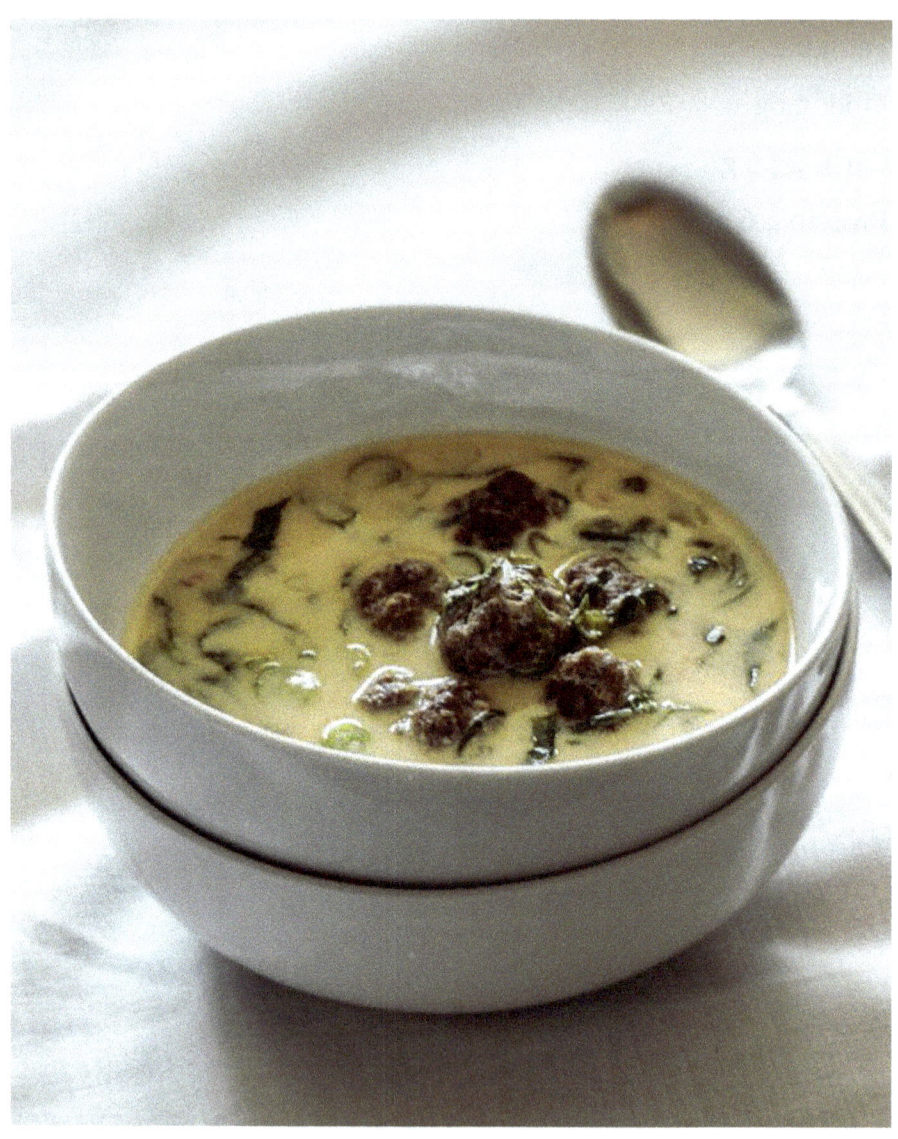

36

Difficulty Level: 2/5

Preparation time: 5 minutes

Cooking time: 20 minutes

Servings: 4

Ingredients

1 lb. Mussels

1 glass White dry wine

8 oz Cheese

8 oz Cream

1/2 Onions head

2 tbsp Olive oil

1 tbsp Parsley, chopped

2 Garlic, cloves

Pepper black ground, to taste

Directions

Chop onions and garlic lightly browned in olive oil. Put the thawed mussels in this mixture, hold them a little on the fire and add the wine.

Wait until the alcohol is half evaporated, add the cheese, parsley and black pepper.

When the cheese melts in the wine, add cream a little bit, bring it to a boil and remove from heat.

Nutrition: (Per serving)

Calories: 115 Kcal

Fat: 7.7 g.

Protein: 6.2 g.

Carbs: 2 g.

Mushroom Cream Soup

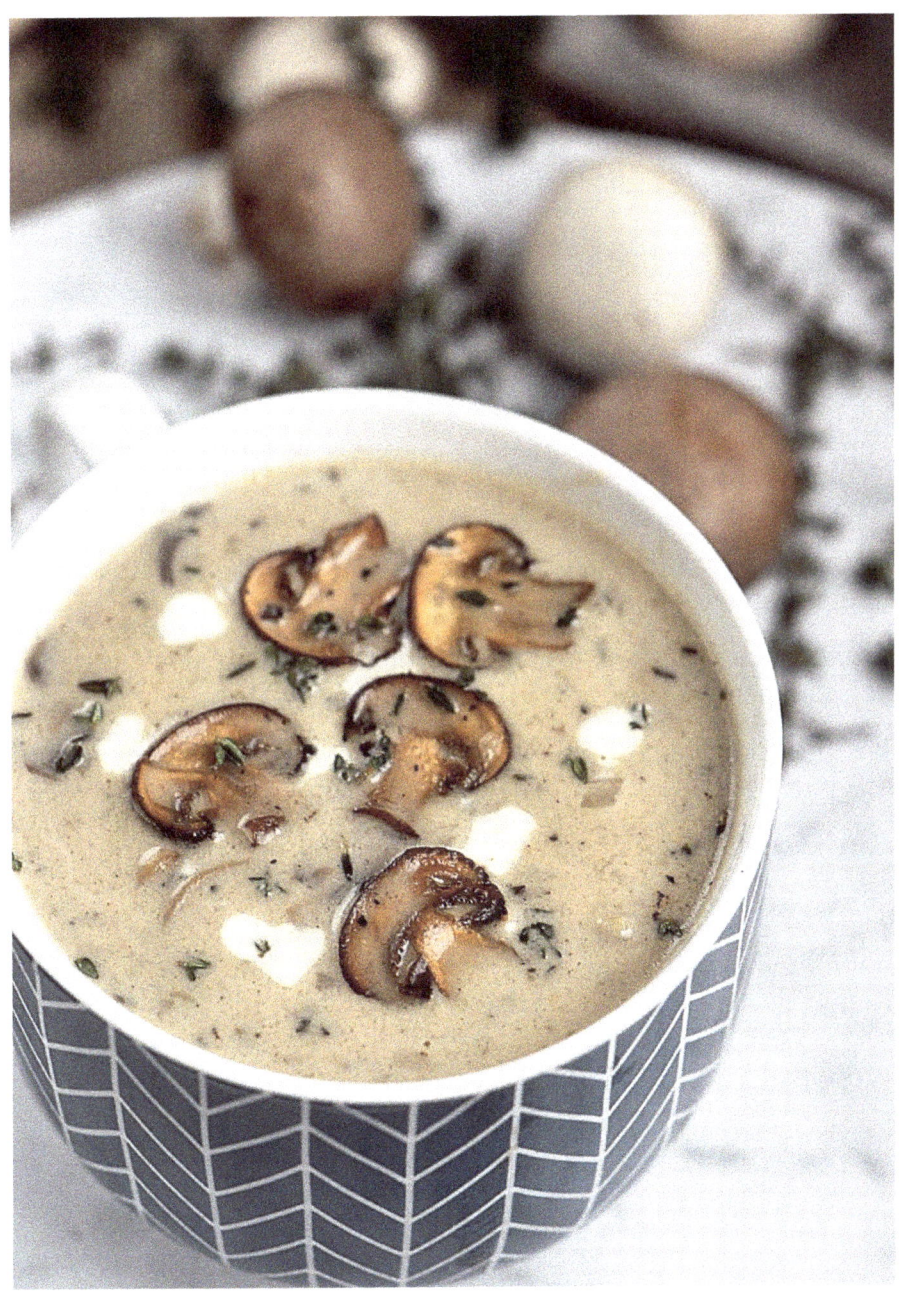

Difficulty Level: 2/5

Preparation time: 5 minutes

Cooking time: 20 minutes

Servings:: 4

Ingredients

1 lb. Champignons

1 lb. Cream 20%

2 Onion

1 oz Butter

Pepper black ground, to taste

Directions

Peel and clean the mushrooms through a meat grinder. Add the finely chopped onion.

Fry the mixture in a pan with olive oil until the water evaporates. Salt and pepper.

Put the fried mushrooms in a saucepan, cover with cream and bring to a boil.

Can be served hot or chilled.

 Nutrition: (Per serving)

Calories: 117 Kcal

Fat: 10.3 g.

Protein: 3.1 g.

Carbs: 3.6 g.

Creamy Salmon Soup

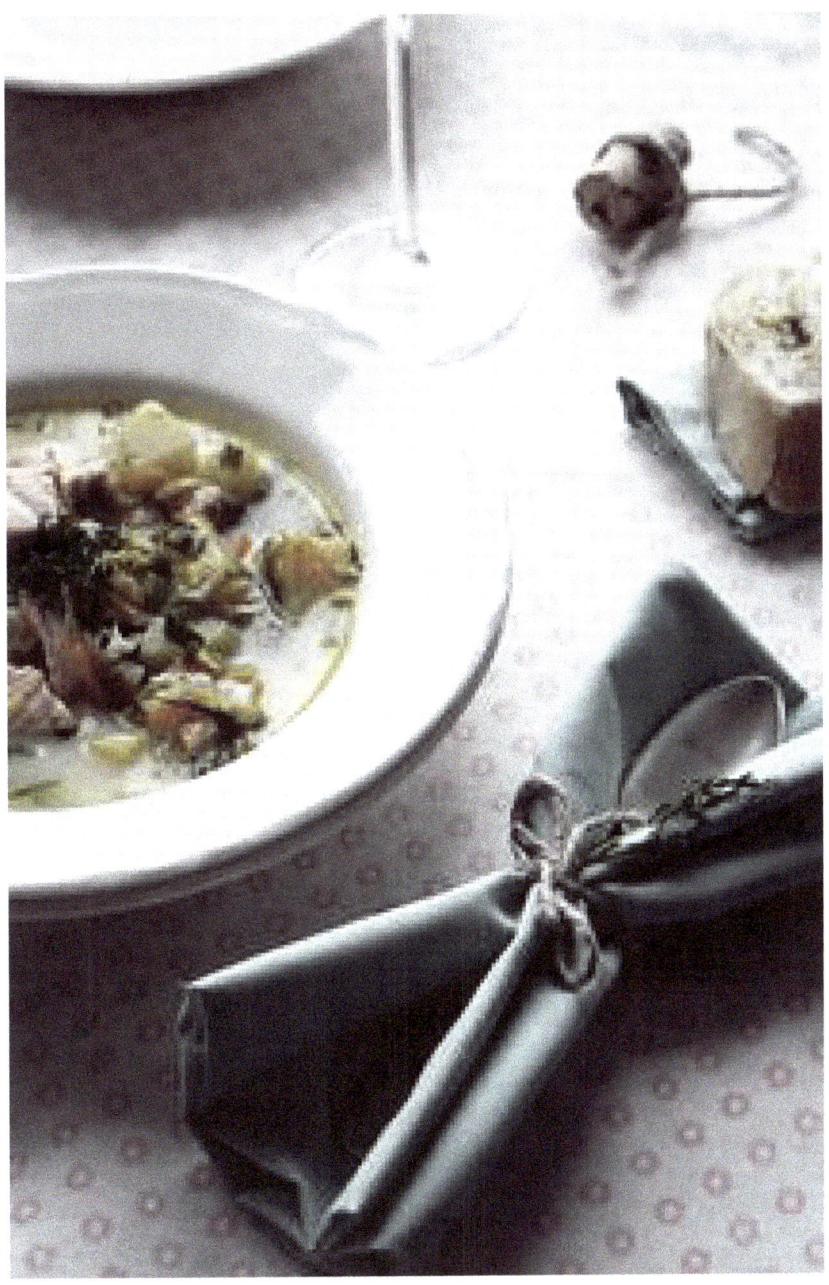

Difficulty Level: 2/5

Preparation time: 5 minutes

Cooking time: 20 minutes

Servings: 6

Ingredients

1 lb. Cream of 10%

1 lb. Potato

11 oz Salmon

10 oz Tomato

7 oz Leek

5 oz Carrot

1 Greens, bunch

2 tbsp Olive Oil

Pepper black ground, to taste

Directions

Cut leek rings, rub carrots with a grater. Peeled potatoes cut into small cubes or cubes. Cut the salmon into cubes.

Peel the tomatoes and cut into cubes. If the skin is badly removed, dip the tomatoes for a few seconds in boiling water.

In a saucepan fry onions and carrots in olive oil. Add tomatoes and fry slightly. Pour 1 liter of water, bring to a boil.

When the water boils, add potatoes, salt to taste, cook for 5-7 minutes. Then add the salmon and pour in the cream. Boil until potatoes are ready (3-5 minutes).

Nutrition: (Per serving)

Calories: 115 Kcal

Fat: 7.7 g.

Protein: 6.2 g.

Carbs: 2 g.

Seafood Salad with Lime Sauce

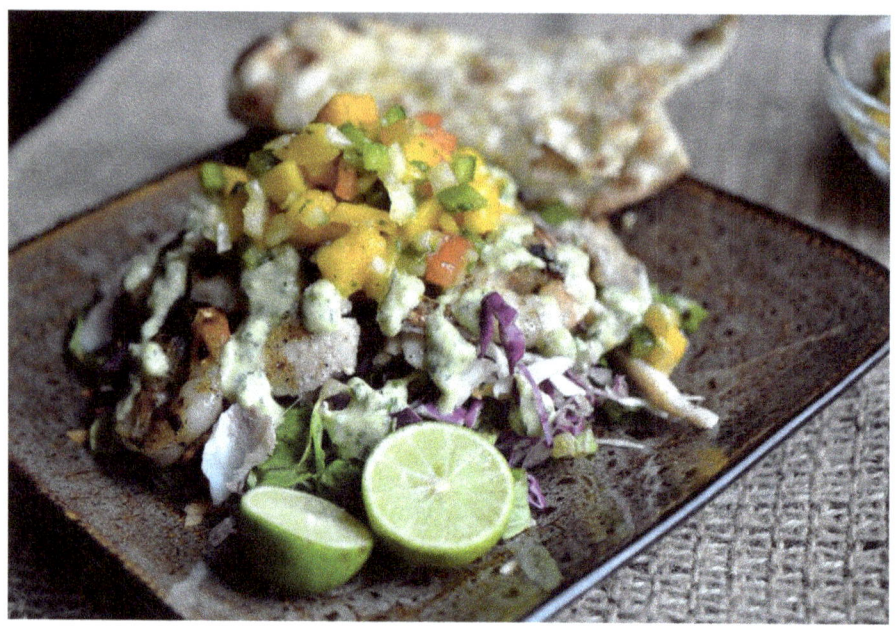

Difficulty Level: 2/5

Preparation time: 5 minutes

Cooking time: 15 minutes

Servings: 2

Ingredients

4 Mussels, pieces

3 Cherry tomatoes

3 oz Cooked shrimp, shredded

2 oz Calamary

2 oz Iceberg lettuce

1/2 Lime

1.5 fl. oz Olive oil

1 oz. Pine nuts

1 tbsp. Cheese Parmesan, grated

Pepper black ground, to taste

Directions

Boil the calamary and cut into strips.

Tear lettuce leaves. Cherry tomatoes cut in half.

Put the pine nuts on a dry frying pan and fry gently all the time, shaking the pan.

Mix the juice of half lime with olive oil, add salt and black pepper to taste.

Put all the ingredients on a plate and pour dressing. Sprinkle with pine nuts on top.

Nutrition: (Per serving)

Calories: 149 Kcal

Fat: 12.2 g.

Protein: 8.1 g.

Carbs: 1.7 g.

Arugula with Radish and Tomatoes

Difficulty Level: 2/5

Preparation time: 5 minutes

Cooking time: 10 minutes

Servings: 2

Ingredients

1 cup Cherry tomatoes

6 Radish, pieces

1 Arugula, bundle

1 tbsp Olive oil

2 tsp Lemon juice

Pepper black ground, to taste

Directions

Wash arugula and tear it into pieces. Radish cut into thin circles. Cherry tomatoes cut in half. Add pine nuts.

Season the mixture with olive oil, lemon juice, salt and pepper to taste.

Nutrition: (Per serving)

Calories: 51 Kcal

Fat: 3.9 g.

Protein: 1.2 g.

Carbs: 2.8 g.

Salad of Colorful Peppers with Basil on The Grill

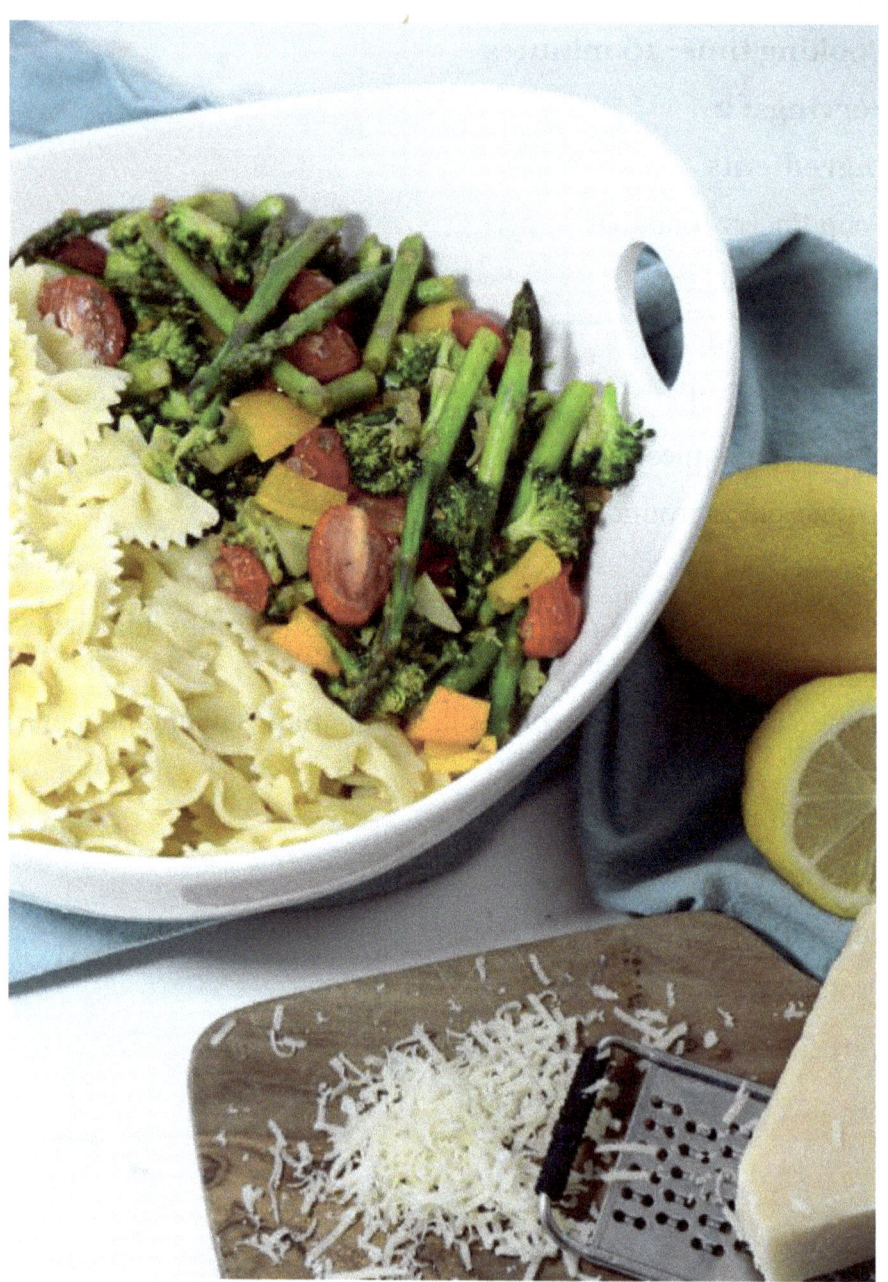

Difficulty Level: 2/5

Preparation time: 5 minutes

Cooking time: 20 minutes

Servings: 4

Ingredients

2 Red bell pepper

2 Yellow bell pepper

2 Green bell pepper

3 Tomato

1/2 cup Basil leaves

1 Onion

5 tbsp Vinegar

4 Olive oil

1 tsp Sugar

1 tsp Salt

Directions

Preheat the grill. Put the peppers on the grill and fry for a few minutes, turning until the skin begins to burn.

Transfer to a bowl, cover with foil and leave for 15 minutes. Peel and peel the skin. Cut into thin strips.

Place the finely chopped onion rings into the microwave container and add sugar, salt, and water so that it completely covers the onion. Microwave for 2 minutes. Drain.

Put peppers, finely chopped tomatoes, and finely chopped basil on a plate. Sprinkle with olive oil and vinegar.

Nutrition: (Per serving)

Calories: 78 Kcal

Fat: 5.7 g.

Protein: 1.2 g.

Carbs: 4.7 g.

Spinach Salad with Pear and Avocado

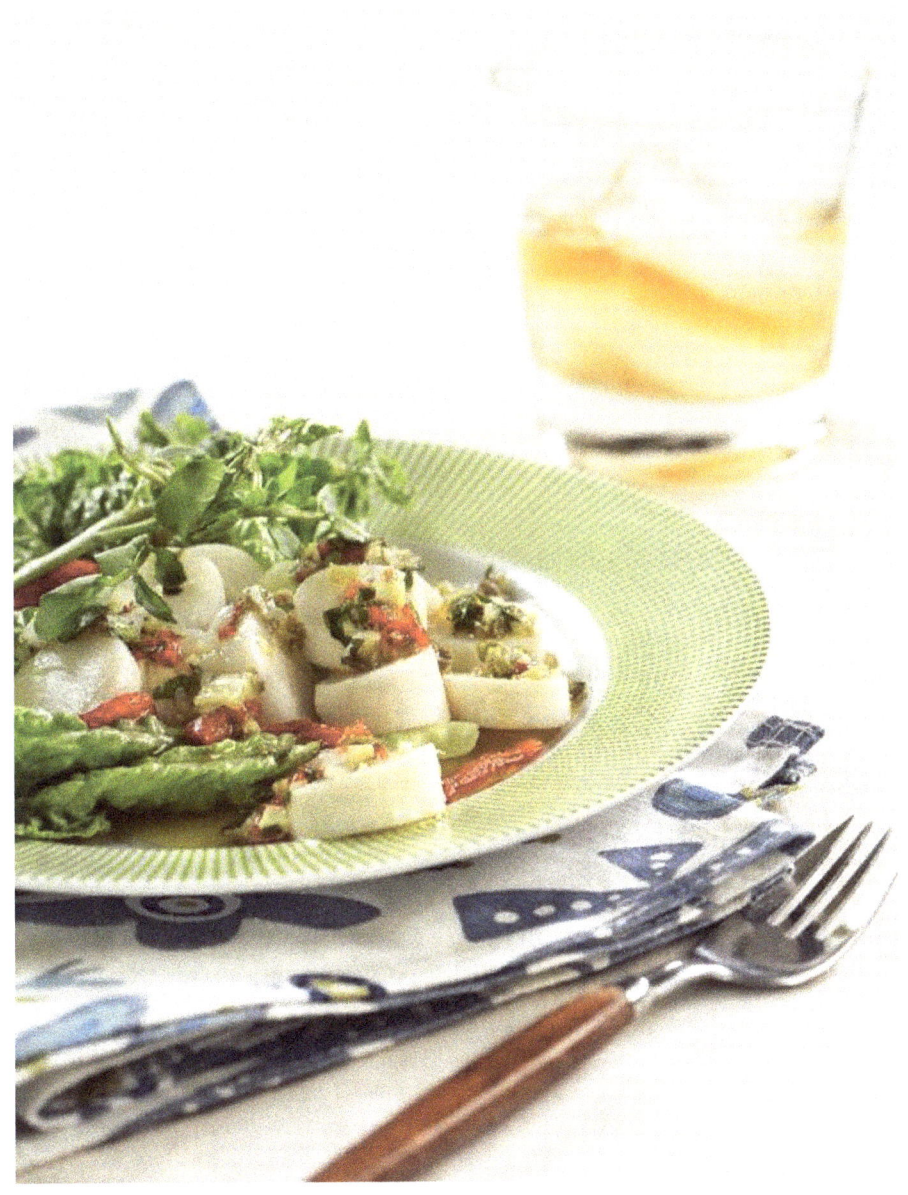

Difficulty Level: 2/5

Preparation time: 5 minutes

Cooking time: 10 minutes

Servings: 2

Ingredients

1 Avocado

1 Pear

6 oz Fresh spinach leaves

4 fl. oz Olive oil

2 fl. oz Rice vinegar

2 oz Gorgonzola Cheese

1/2 red onion

1 tbsp Cilantro, chopped

1 tbsp Lime juice

Cayenne pepper, to taste

1/4 tsp Ground dried garlic

Directions

In a small bowl, mix the olive oil, vinegar, lime juice, cilantro, garlic, and cayenne pepper. Salt and pepper.

In another larger bowl, gently mix the spinach, diced pear, finely chopped avocado, and finely chopped onion.

Pour over the dressing, stir and sprinkle with cheese. Serve with the remaining dressing.

Nutrition: (Per serving)

Calories: 210 Kcal

Fat: 19.6 g.

Protein: 2.5 g.
Carbs: 6.7 g.

Cherry Tomato Salad with Shrimps

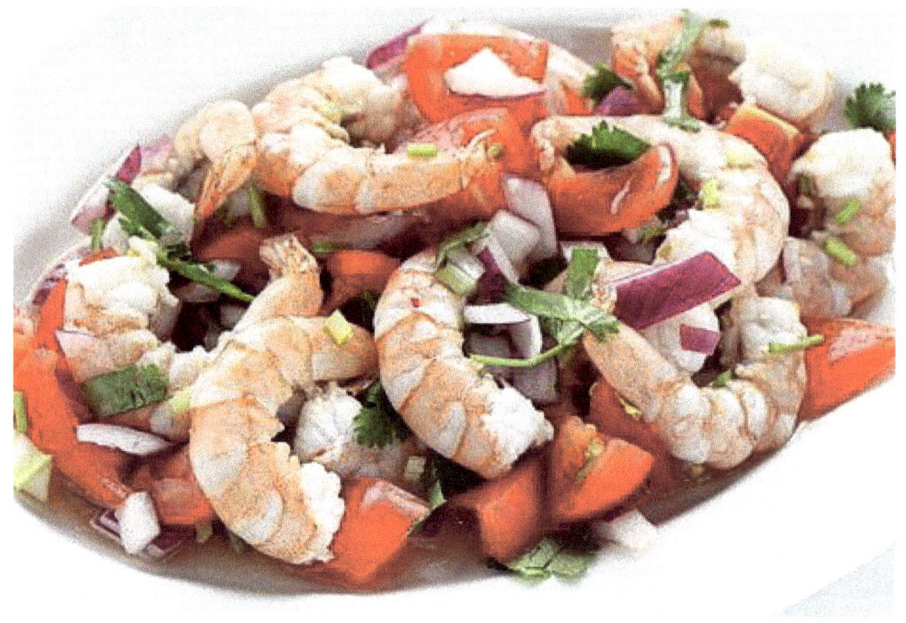

Difficulty Level: 2/5
Preparation time: 5 minutes
Cooking time: 10 minutes
Servings: 2
Ingredients

11 oz Cherry tomato

4 oz Boiled shrimps, peeled

1oz Green basil

1 fl. oz Olive oil

lb. Mussels

1 glass White dry wine

8 oz Cheese

8 oz Cream

1/2 Onions head

2 tbsp Olive oil

1 tbsp Parsley, chopped

2 Garlic, cloves

Pepper black ground, to taste

Directions

Cherry tomatoes cut in half and add peeled shrimp.

Add the chopped basil leaves.

Add olive oil, add salt and pepper.

Nutrition: (Per serving)

Calories: 66 Kcal

Fat: 4.9 g.

Protein: 3.8 g.
Carbs: 2.1 g.

Green Salad with Cherry and Pine Nuts

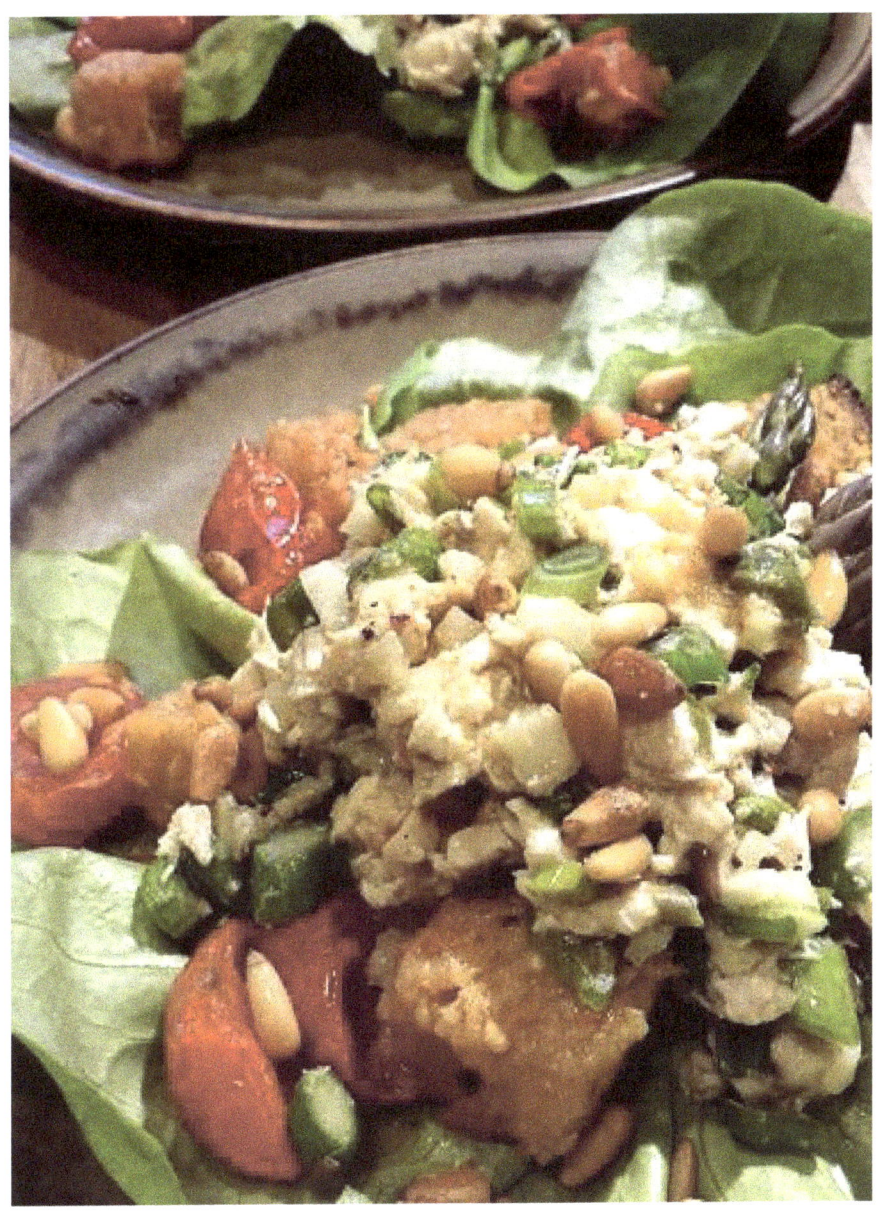

Difficulty Level: 2/5

Preparation time: 5 minutes

Cooking time: 10 minutes

Servings: 2

Ingredients

1.5 cup Romano Salad

1.5 cup Arugula

10 Cherry tomato

2 tbsp Pine nuts

2 tbsp Olive oil

1.5 Lime juice

1/2 Garlic, clove

Sea salt, pinch

Parmesan, to taste

Pepper black ground, to taste

Directions

Mix lemon juice, olive oil, chopped garlic, salt and pepper.

In another container, mix lettuce, arugula, cherry halves and drizzle with dressing.

Stir and sprinkle with nuts and parmesan on top - to taste.

Nutrition: (Per serving)

Calories: 66 Kcal

Fat: 5.3 g.

Protein: 1.9 g.

Carbs: 2.6 g.

Shopsky Salad

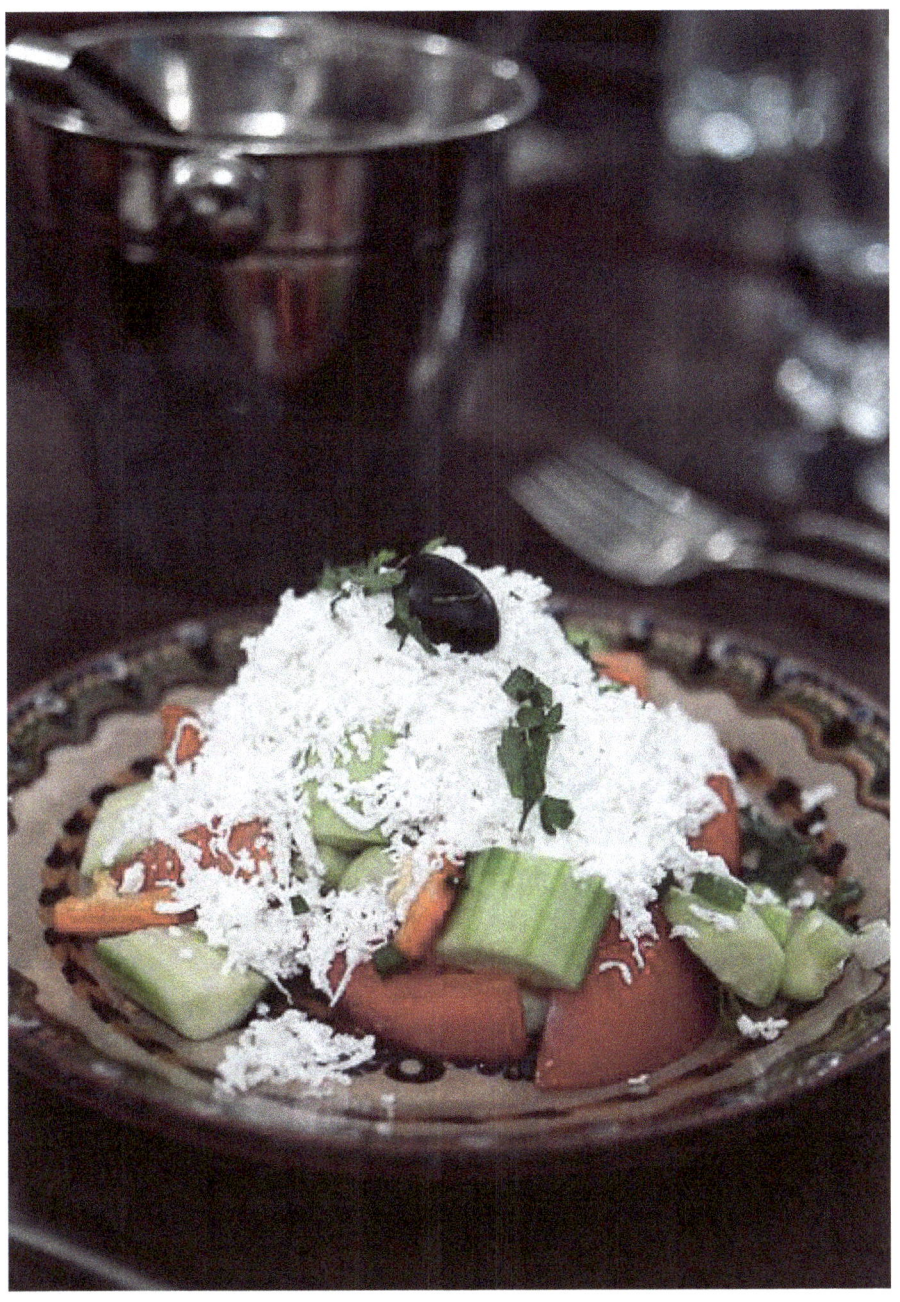

Difficulty Level: 2/5

Preparation time: 5 minutes

Cooking time: 20 minutes

Servings: 4

Ingredients

1 lb. Bell pepper

11 oz Tomato

5 oz Cucumber

5 oz White cheese

1 Chili pepper

4 oz Onion

2 fl. oz Olive oil

Parsley, chopped, to taste

Vinegar, to taste

Directions

Fry the peppers in the oven until the skin is slightly browned. Remove the peel and seeds, and then cut the pepper into small pieces.

Cut the tomatoes and cucumbers into small pieces. Onions cut into thin half rings. Put the vegetables in a bowl and mix. Add salt to taste, then butter and parsley. Mix well again and place on the dish.

Sprinkle with grated cheese and garnish with finely chopped chili.

Nutrition: (Per serving)

Calories: 91 Kcal

Fat: 3 g.

Protein: 6.2 g.

Carbs: 4.7 g.

Spinach Salad

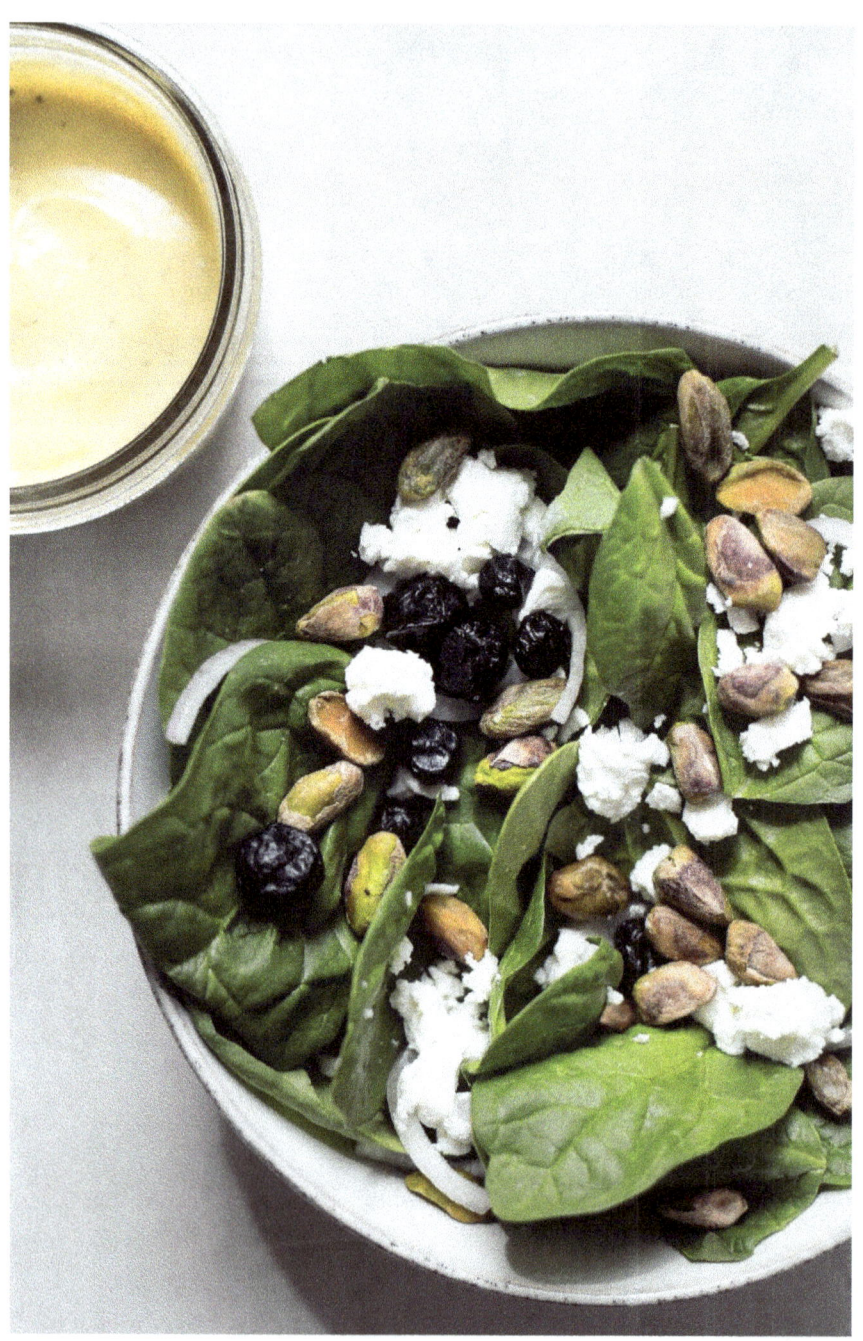

Difficulty Level: 2/5

Preparation time: 5 minutes

Cooking time: 10 minutes

Servings: 2

Ingredients

1 Spinach, bundle

2 tbsp Lemon juice

2 tbsp Walnut

1 tsp Soy sauce

1 Garlic, clove

Pepper black ground, to taste

Directions

Scrub the washed spinach with boiling water and rinse under cold water.

Mix lemon juice and soy sauce, add walnuts and squeeze garlic cloves. Mix everything thoroughly, dressing the spinach leaves.

Nutrition: (Per serving)

Calories: 155 Kcal

Fat: 13.7 g.

Protein: 5.2 g.

Carbs: 4 g.

Seasonal Salad with Red Bean, Curd Cheese, and Red Onion

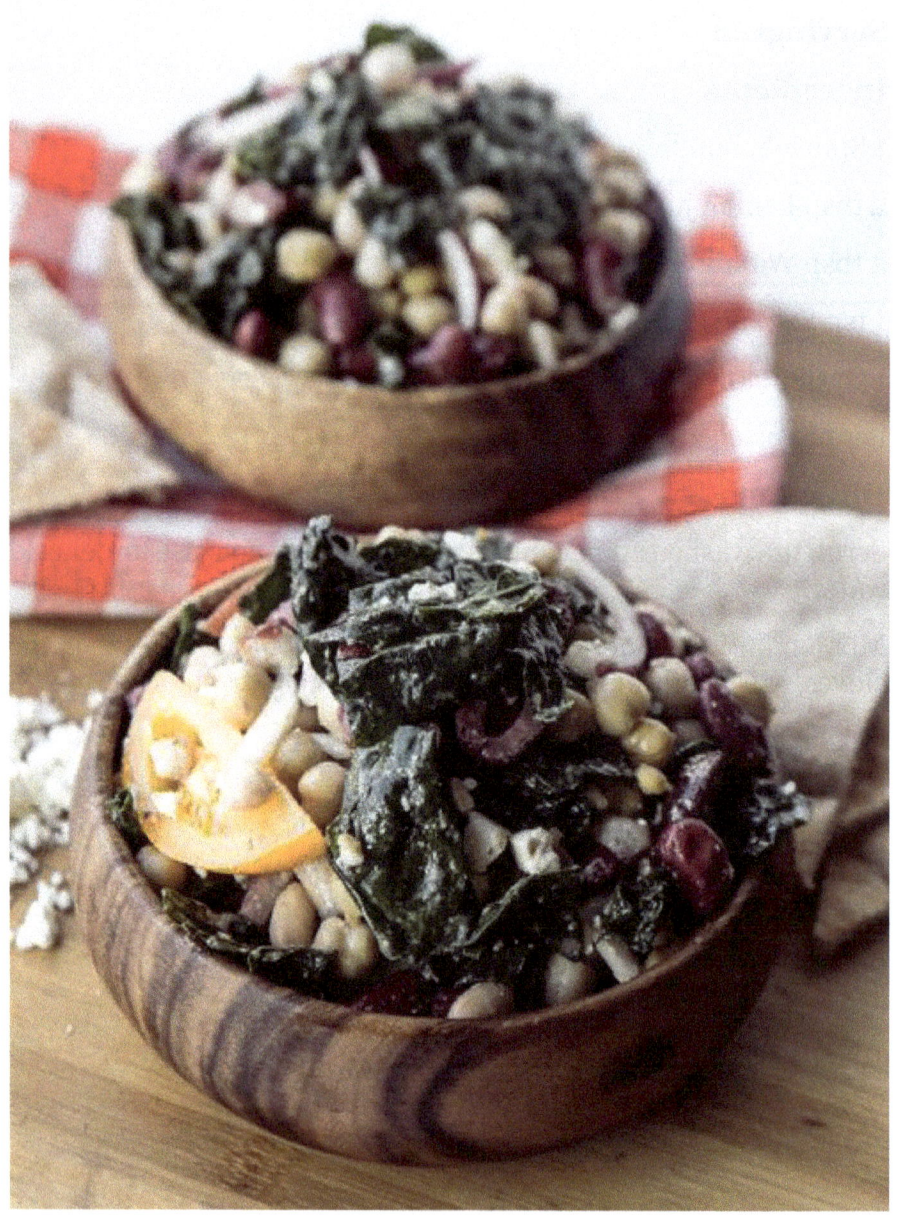

Difficulty Level: 1/5

Preparation time: 7 minutes

Cooking time: 0 minutes

Servings: 4

Ingredients

1 lb. Canned Beans

7 oz Cheese curd

1 Limon

4 oz Arugula

2 fl. oz Olive oil

2 oz Red onion

2 Garlic, cloves

Pepper black ground, to taste

Directions

Take two cans of red beans, drain the juice from it and rinse with cold water.

Mix the beans with finely chopped red onions, herbs, garlic, olive oil, lemon juice, and curd cheese.

Salt, pepper and leave to mix.

Nutrition: (Per serving)

Calories: 134 Kcal

Fat: 7.6 g.

Protein: 7.1 g.

Carbs: 9 g.

Green Bean and Cherry Salad with Shallot

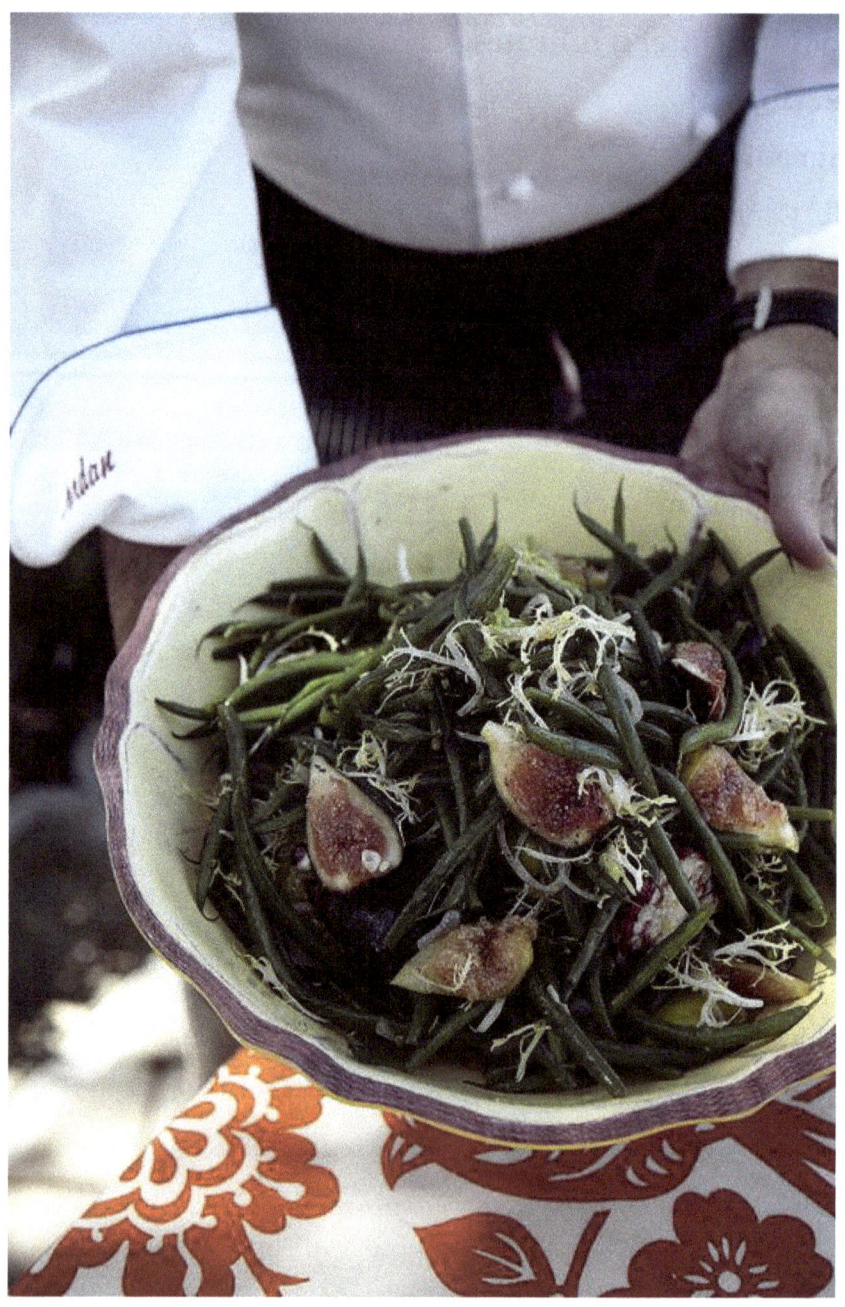

Difficulty Level: 2/5

Preparation time: 5 minutes

Cooking time: 10 minutes

Servings: 4

Ingredients

1 lb. Green String Beans

1 lb. Red cherry tomato

6 tbsp Olive oil

2 tbsp Red wine vinegar

1 Onion

Basil leave, to taste

Pepper black ground, to taste

Directions

Cut off the tails of the beans and cut into small pieces. Put in a pot of boiling salted water and boil until soft for about 5 minutes.

Put on ice or rinse under cold water. Dry and transfer to a bowl. Cut the cherry in half and place in another bowl.

Chop the onion and place in a small bowl. Add vinegar, salt, and pepper. Add to the cherry and mix well.

Before serving, mix with beans and basil.

Nutrition: (Per serving)

Calories: 88 Kcal

Fat: 7.7 g.

Protein: 2.1 g.

Carbs: 3.2 g.

Easy Shrimp Salad

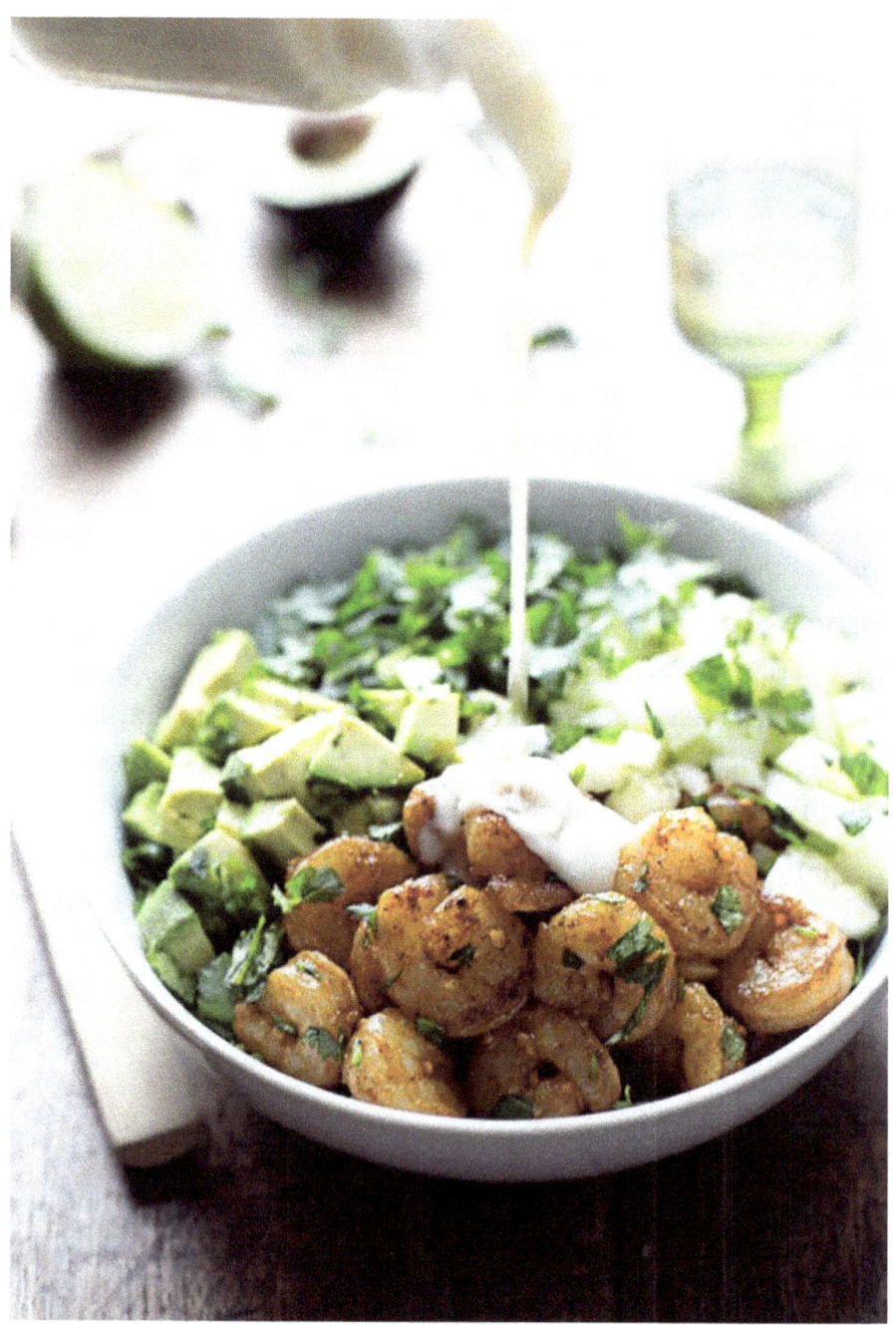

Difficulty Level: 2/5

Preparation time: 5 minutes

Cooking time: 10 minutes

Servings: 4

Ingredients

1 lb. Shrimps

5 oz Green Salad

5 oz Cherry tomato

4 oz Arugula

4 tbsp Olive oil

4 tbsp Limon juice

2 tbsp Dry white wine

2 tbsp Soy sauce

Pepper black ground, to taste

Directions

Put shrimp in boiling salted water and cook for 3 minutes. Flip down, rinse with cold water and clean. Slightly fry the shrimps in olive oil, then pour them with lemon juice and soy sauce and let stand for a while.

Cut the cherry tomatoes into two halves, pickle the lettuce leaves and add the shrimps, previously draining the liquid from them.

Refill the remaining lemon juice, soy sauce, olive oil, and wine. Pepper, salt to taste and pour the salad with the resulting sauce.

Nutrition: (Per serving)

Calories: 117 Kcal

Fat: 7.6 g.

Protein: 10.3 g.

Carbs: 1.2 g.

Healthy Vegetable Soup

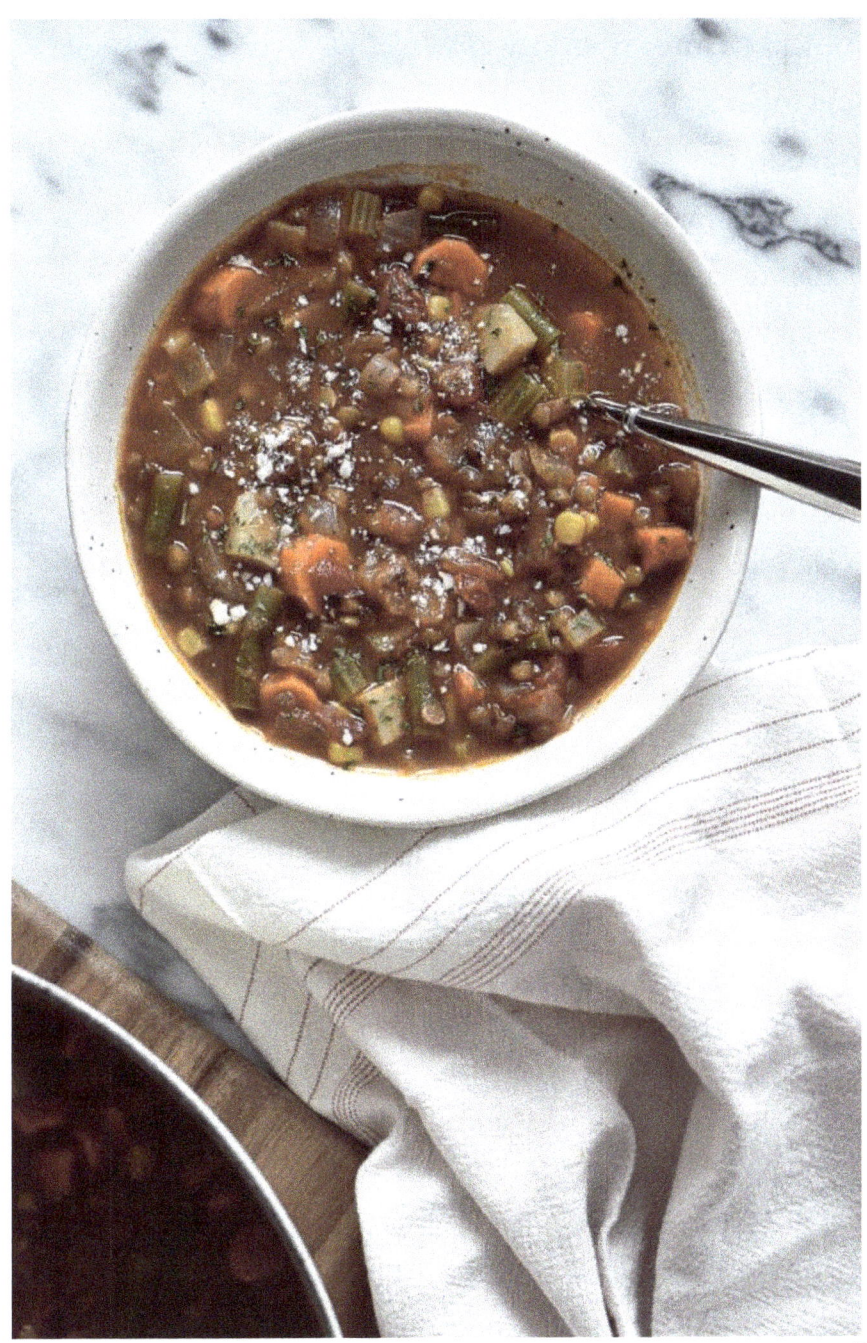

Difficulty Level: 2/5

Preparation Time: 10 minutes

Cooking Time: 15 minutes

Servings: 4

Ingredients:

1 cup can tomatoes, chopped

1 small zucchini, diced

3 oz kale, sliced

1 tbsp garlic, chopped

5 button mushrooms, sliced

2 carrots, peeled and sliced

2 celery sticks, sliced

1/2 red chili, sliced

1 onion, diced

1 tbsp olive oil

1 bay leaf

4 cups vegetable stock

1/4 tsp salt

Directions:

Add oil into the inner pot of Pressure Pot and set the pot on sauté mode.

Add carrots, celery, onion, and salt and cook for 2-3 minutes.

Add mushrooms and chili and cook for 2 minutes.

Add remaining ingredients and stir everything well.

Seal pot with lid and cook on high for 10 minutes.

Once done, allow to release pressure naturally for 10 minutes then release remaining using quick release. Remove lid.

Stir well and serve.

Nutrition: (Per serving)

Calories 100

Fat 3.8 g

Carbohydrates 15.1 g

Sugar 6.6 g

Protein 3.5 g

Cholesterol 0 mg

Delicious Okra Chicken Stew

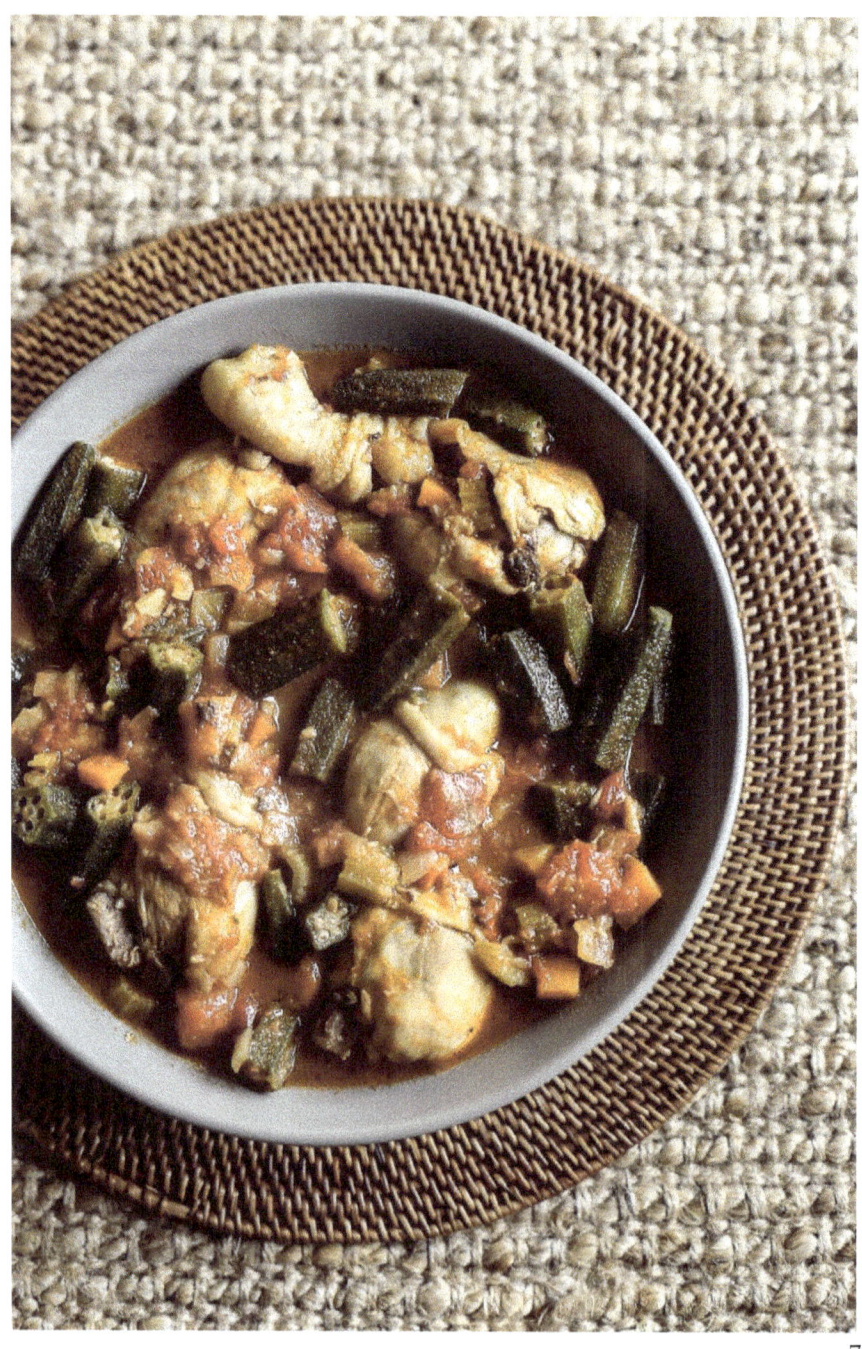

Difficulty Level: 2/5

Preparation Time: 10 minutes

Cooking Time: 20 minutes

Servings: 4

Ingredients:

1 lb chicken breasts, skinless, boneless, and cubed

1 lemon juice

1/4 cup fresh parsley, chopped

1 tbsp olive oil

12 oz can tomatoes, crushed

1 tsp allspice

14 oz okra, chopped

2 cups chicken stock

1 tsp garlic, minced

1 onion, chopped

Pepper

Salt

Directions:

Add oil into the inner pot of Pressure Pot and set the pot on sauté mode.

Add chicken and onion and sauté until chicken is lightly brown about 5 minutes.

Add remaining ingredients except for the parsley and stir well.

Seal pot with lid and cook on high pressure 15 for minutes.

Once done, allow to release pressure naturally for 10 minutes then release remaining using quick release. Remove lid.

Stir well and serve.

Nutrition: (Per serving)

Calories 326

Fat 12.6 g

Carbohydrates 15.8 g

Sugar 6.2 g

Protein 36.4 g

Cholesterol 101 mg

Garlic Squash Broccoli Soup

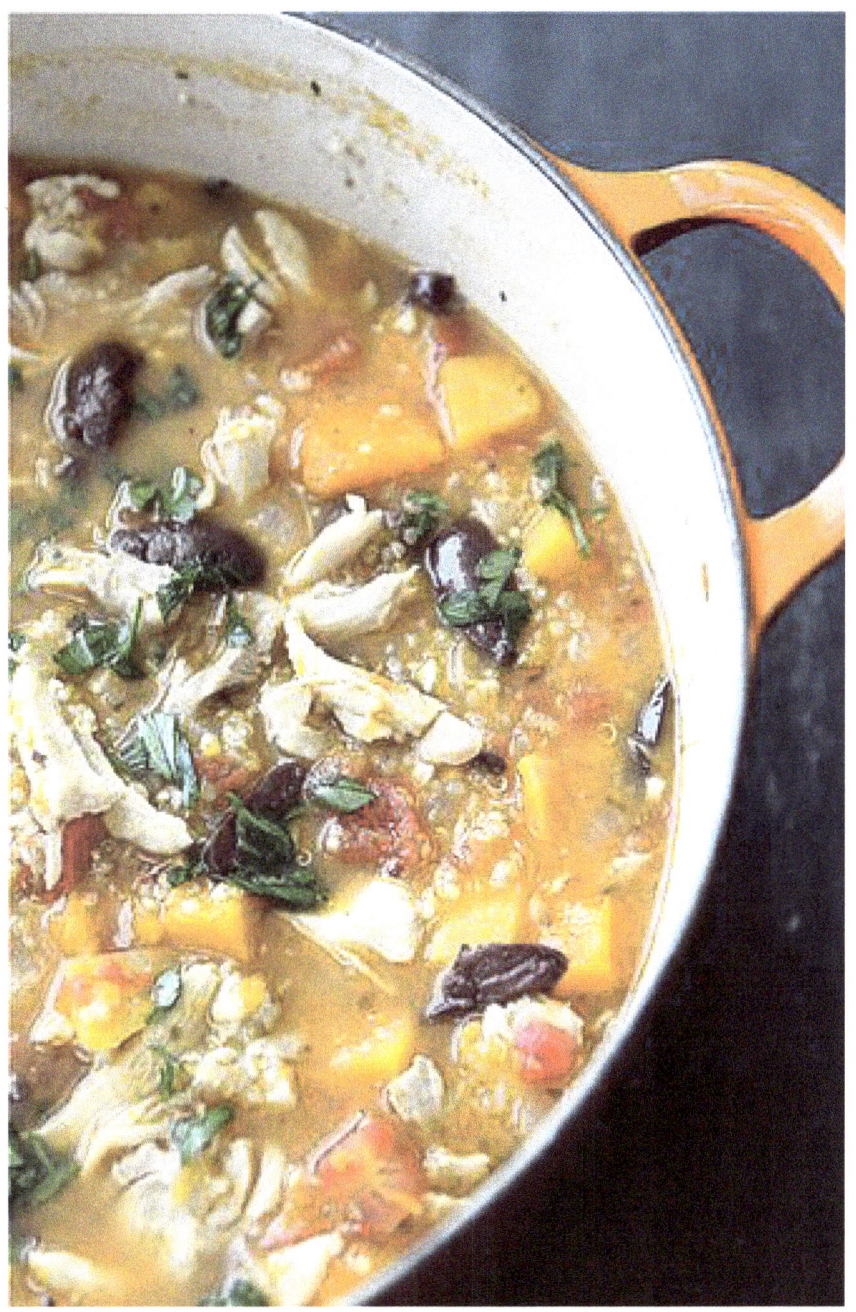

Preparation Time: 10 minutes

Cooking Time: 15 minutes

Servings: 4

Ingredients:

1 lb butternut squash, peeled and diced

1 lb broccoli florets

1 tsp dried basil

1 tsp paprika

2 1/2 cups vegetable stock

1 tsp garlic, minced

1 tbsp olive oil

1 onion, chopped

Salt

Directions:

Add oil into the inner pot of Pressure Pot and set the pot on sauté mode.

Add onion and garlic and sauté for 3 minutes.

Add remaining ingredients and stir well.

Seal pot with lid and cook on high pressure 12 for minutes.

Once done, allow to release pressure naturally for 10 minutes then release remaining using quick release. Remove lid.

Blend soup using an immersion blender until smooth.

Serve and enjoy.

Nutrition: (Per serving)

Calories 137

Fat 4.1 g

Carbohydrates 24.5 g

Sugar 6.1 g

Protein 5 g

Cholesterol 0 mg

Chicken Rice Soup

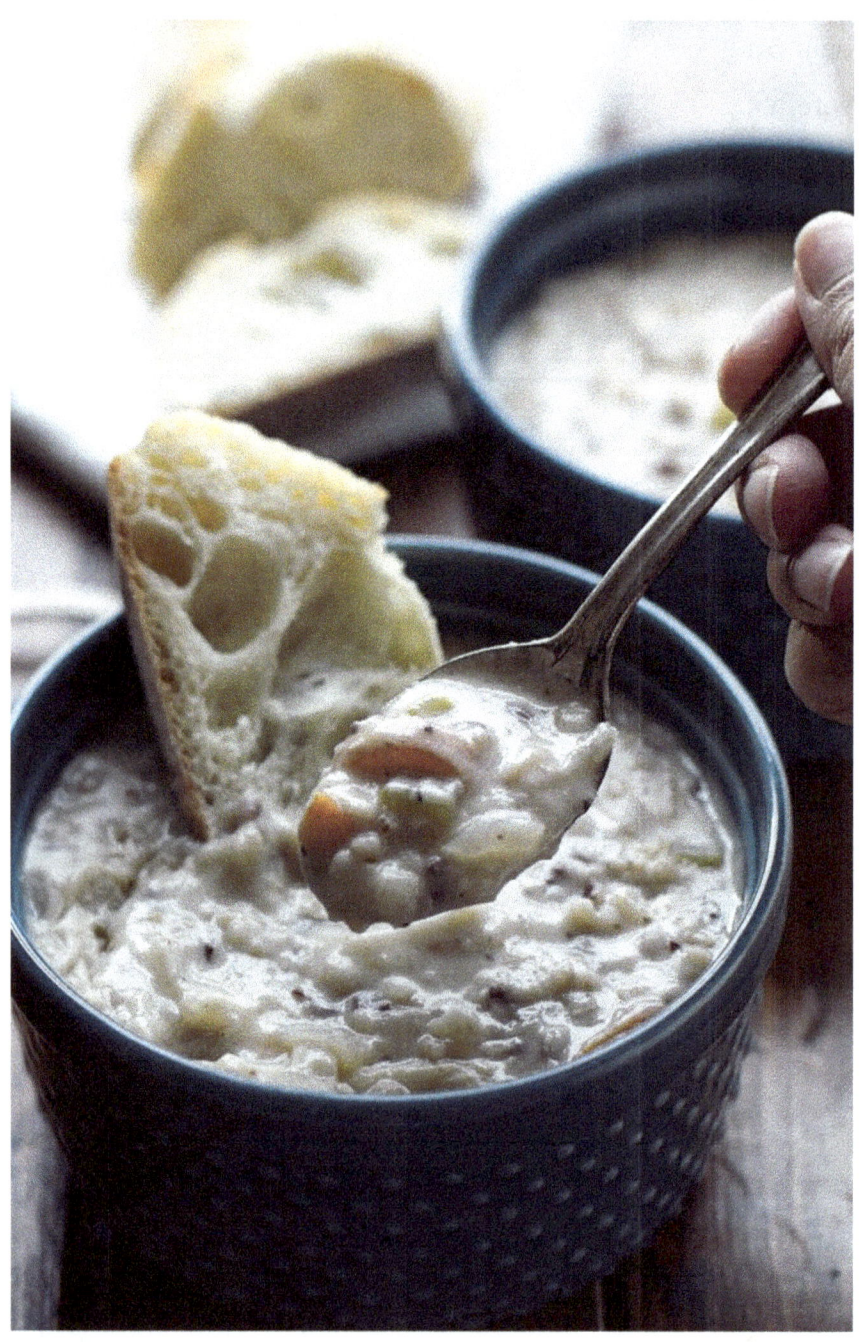

Difficulty Level: 2/5

Preparation Time: 10 minutes

Cooking Time: 9 minutes

Servings: 4

Ingredients:

1 lb chicken breast, boneless

2 thyme sprigs

1 tsp garlic, chopped

1/4 tsp turmeric

1 tbsp olive oil

2 tbsp fresh parsley, chopped

2 tbsp fresh lemon juice

1/4 cup rice

1/2 cup celery, diced

1/2 cup onion, chopped

2 carrots, chopped

5 cups vegetable stock

Pepper

Salt

Directions:

Add oil into the inner pot of Pressure Pot and set the pot on sauté mode.

Add garlic, onion, carrots, and celery and sauté for 3 minutes.

Add the rest of the ingredients and stir well.

Seal pot with lid and cook on high for 6 minutes.

Once done, release pressure using quick release. Remove lid.

Shred chicken using a fork.

Serve and enjoy.

Nutrition: (Per serving)

Calories 237

Fat 6.8 g

Carbohydrates 16.6 g

Sugar 3.4 g

Protein 26.2 g

Cholesterol 73 mg

Mussels Soup

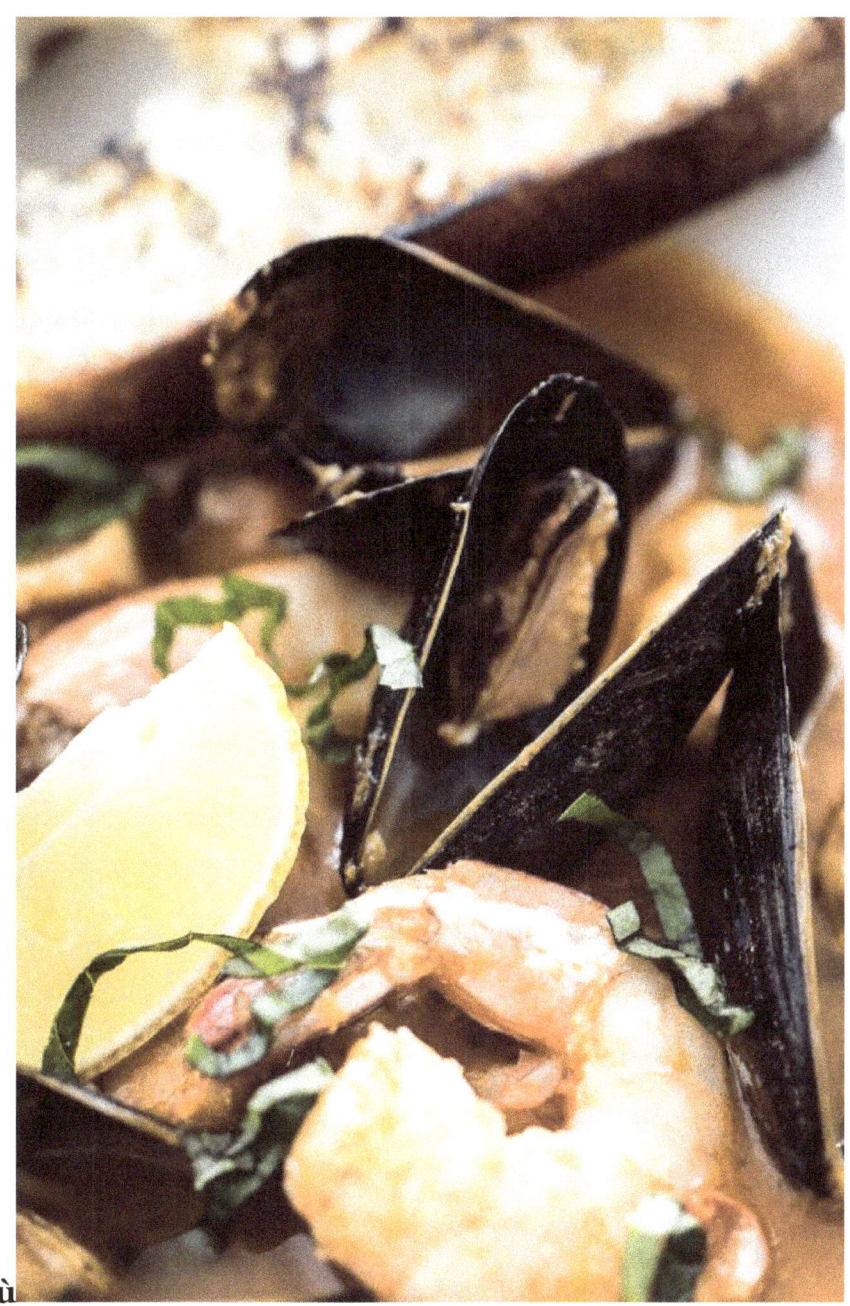

Difficulty Level: 2/5

Preparation Time: 10 minutes

Cooking Time: 3 minutes

Servings: 2

Ingredients:

6 oz mussels, cleaned

2 tsp Italian seasoning

2 tbsp olive oil

1 cup grape tomatoes, chopped

4 cups chicken stock

1/4 cup fish sauce

Directions:

Add all ingredients into the inner pot of Pressure Pot and stir well.

Seal pot with lid and cook on high for 3 minutes.

Once done, release pressure using quick release. Remove lid.

Stir well and serve.

Nutrition: (Per serving)

Calories 256

Fat 18.6 g

Carbohydrates 9.9 g

Sugar 5.5 g

Protein 14.1 g

Cholesterol 27 mg

Creamy Chicken Soup

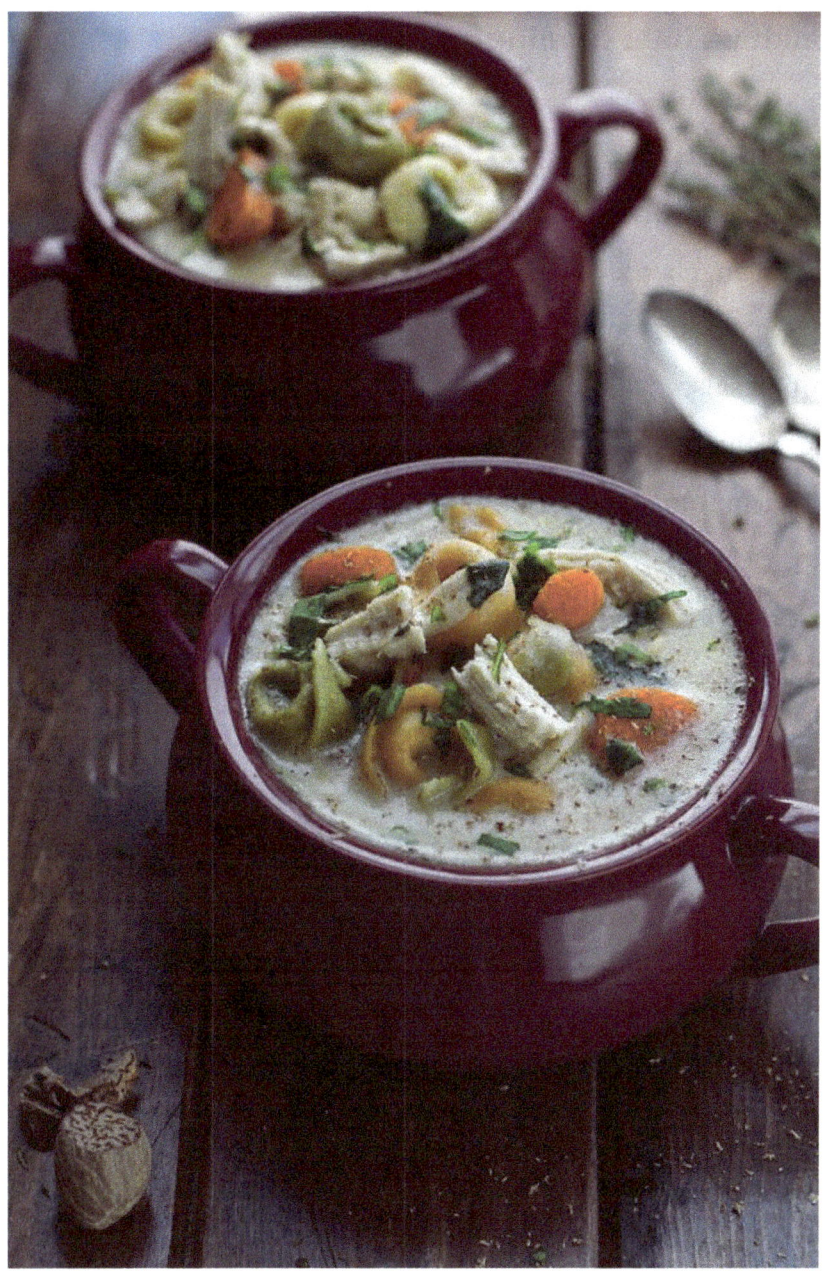

Difficulty Level: 2/5

Preparation Time: 10 minutes

Cooking Time: 10 minutes

Servings: 6

Ingredients:

2 lbs chicken breast, boneless and cut into chunks

8 oz cream cheese

2 tbsp taco seasoning

1 cup of salsa

2 cups chicken stock

28 oz can tomatoes, diced

Salt

Directions:

Add all ingredients except cream cheese into the Pressure Pot.

Seal pot with lid and cook on high pressure 10 for minutes.

Once done, allow to release pressure naturally. Remove lid.

Remove chicken from pot and shred using a fork. Return shredded chicken to the pot.

Add cream cheese and stir well.

Serve and enjoy.

Nutrition: (Per serving)

Calories 471

Fat 24.1 g

Carbohydrates 19.6 g

Sugar 6.2 g

Protein 43.9 g

Cholesterol 157 mg

Cheesy Chicken Soup

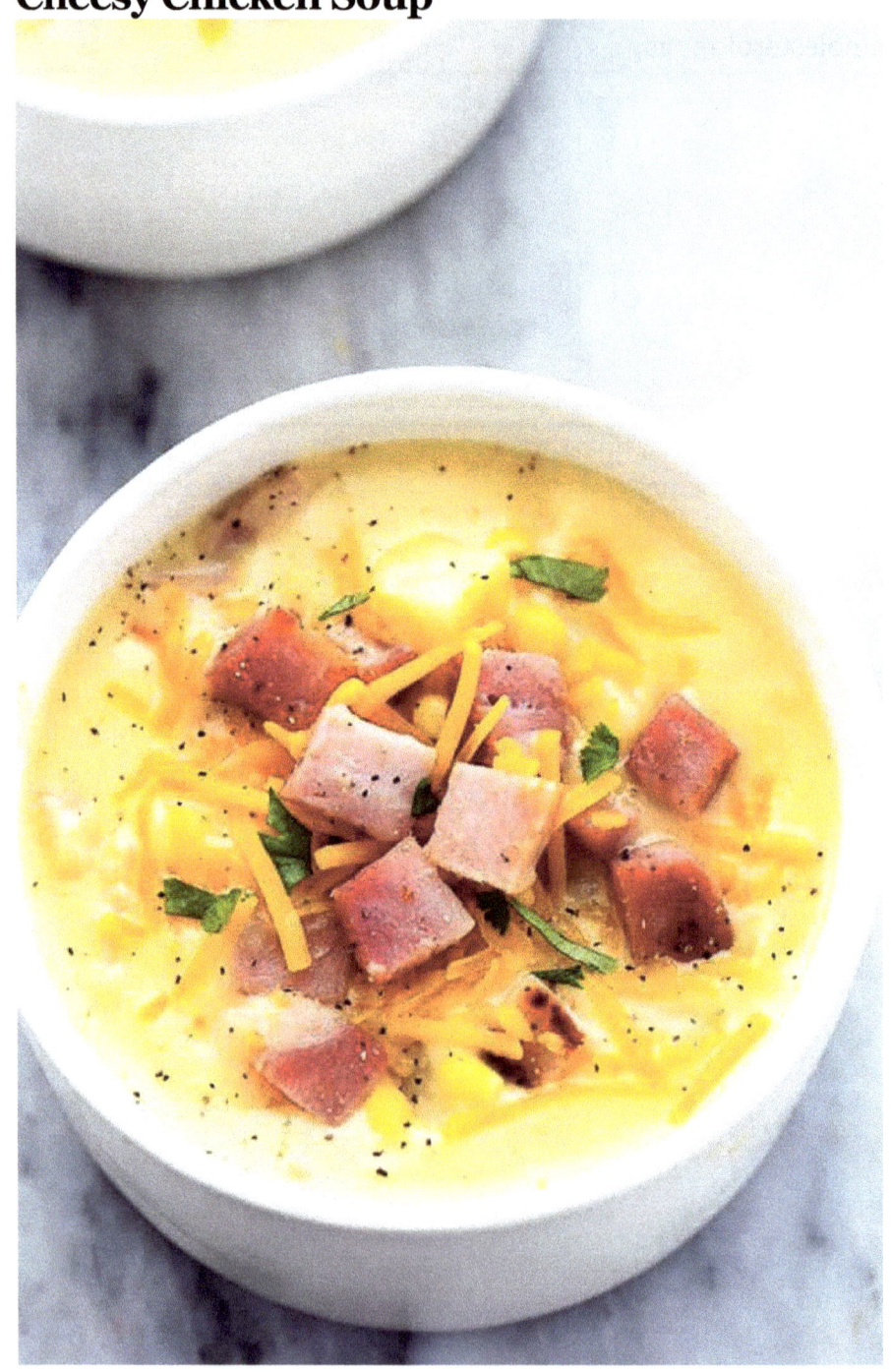

Difficulty Level: 2/5
Preparation Time: 10 minutes
Cooking Time: 15 minutes
Servings: 4
Ingredients:

12 oz chicken thighs, boneless

1 cup heavy cream

2 cups cheddar cheese, shredded

3 cups chicken stock

2 tbsp olive oil

1/2 cup celery, chopped

1/4 cup hot sauce

1 tsp garlic, minced

1/4 cup onion, chopped

Directions:

Add all ingredients except cream and cheese into the Pressure Pot and stir well.

Seal pot with lid and cook on high pressure 15 for minutes.

Once done, allow to release pressure naturally. Remove lid.

Shred the chicken using a fork.

Add cream and cheese and stir until cheese is melted.

Serve and enjoy.

Nutrition: (Per serving)

Calories 568

Fat 43.6 g

Carbohydrates 3.6 g

Sugar 1.5 g

Protein 40.1 g

Cholesterol 176 mg

Italian Chicken Stew

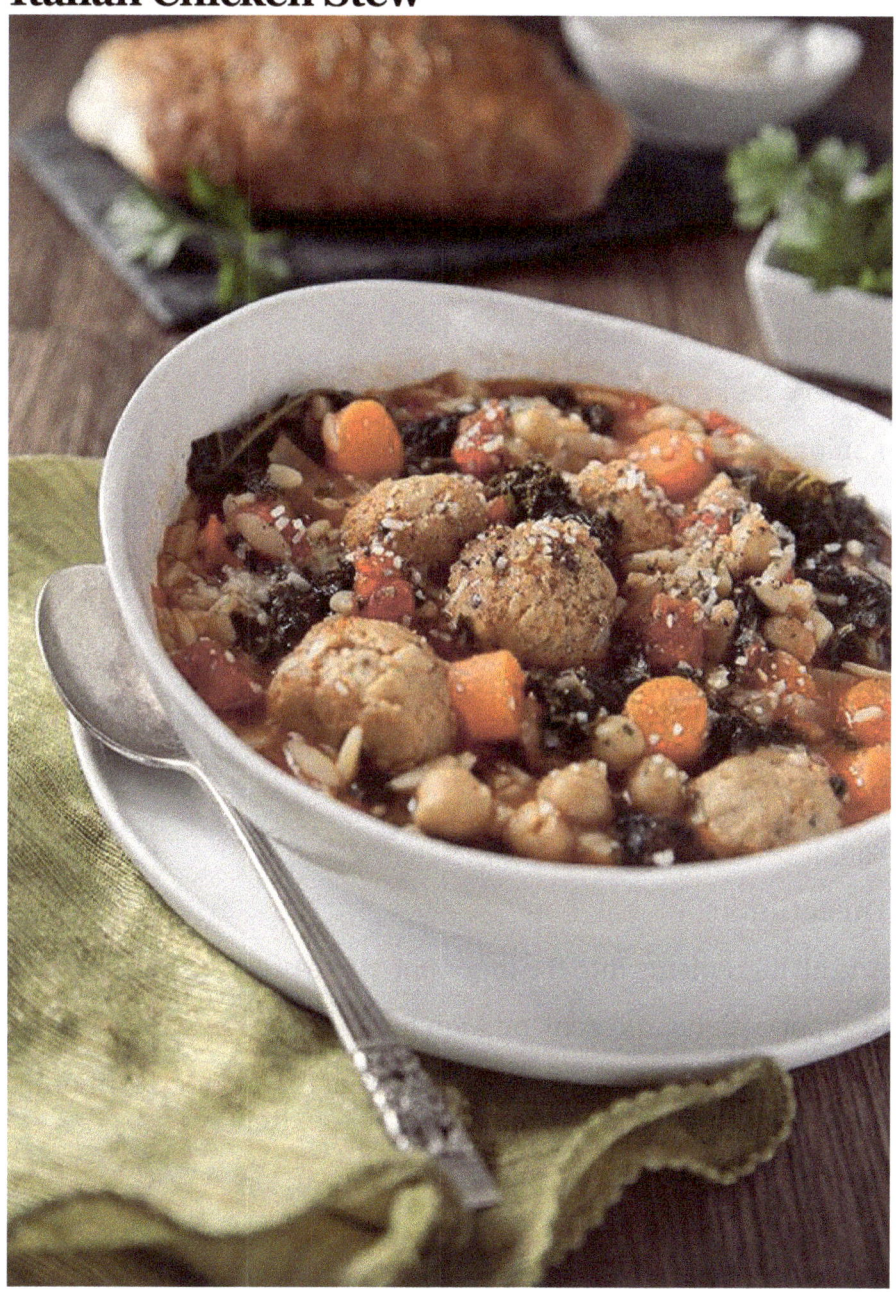

Difficulty Level: 2/5

Preparation Time: 10 minutes

Cooking Time: 12 minutes

Servings: 6

Ingredients:

1 lb chicken breasts, boneless

2 potatoes, peeled and diced

3 carrots, cut into chunks

2 celery stalks, cut into chunks

1 onion, diced

1 tsp garlic, minced

1 tsp ground sage

1/2 tsp thyme

1/2 tsp dried basil

3 cups chicken stock

Pepper

Salt

Directions:

Add all ingredients into the inner pot of Pressure Pot and stir well.

Seal pot with lid and cook on high for 12 minutes.

Once done, allow to release pressure naturally for 10 minutes then release remaining using quick release. Remove lid.

Remove chicken from pot and shred using a fork. Return shredded chicken to the pot.

Stir well and serve.

Nutrition: (Per serving)

Calories 220

Fat 6 g

Carbohydrates 16.7 g

Sugar 3.5 g

Protein 23.9 g

Cholesterol 67 mg

Creamy Carrot Tomato Soup

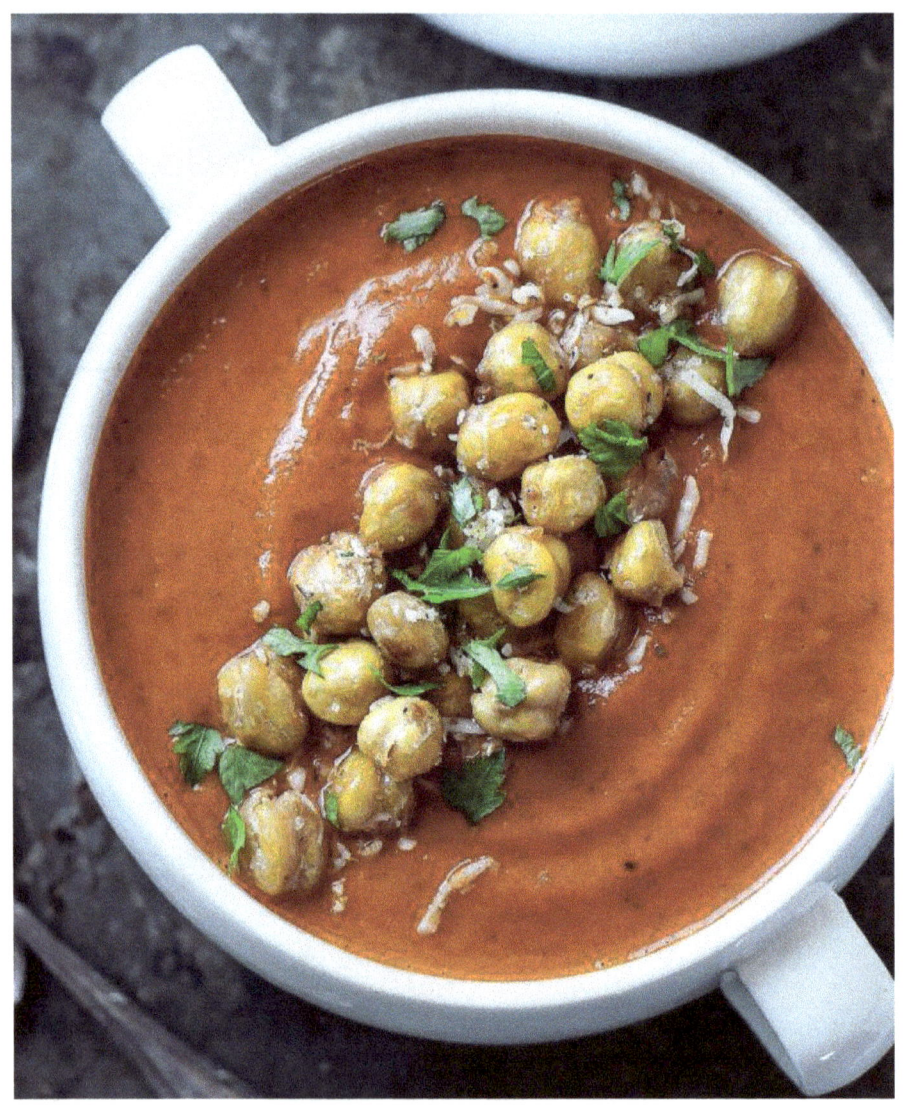

Difficulty Level: 2/5

Preparation Time: 10 minutes

Cooking Time: 10 minutes

Servings: 6

Ingredients:

4 oz can tomatoes, diced

1/2 cup heavy cream

1 cup vegetable broth

1 tbsp dried basil

1 onion, chopped

4 large carrots, peeled and chopped

1/4 cup olive oil

Pepper

Salt

Directions:

Add oil into the inner pot of Pressure Pot and set the pot on sauté mode.

Add onion and carrots and sauté for 5 minutes.

Add the rest of ingredients except heavy cream and stir well.

Seal pot with lid and cook on high pressure 5 for minutes.

Once done, allow to release pressure naturally. Remove lid.

Stir in heavy cream and blend soup using an immersion blender until smooth.

Serve and enjoy.

Nutrition: (Per serving)

Calories 144

Fat 12.4 g

Carbohydrates 7.8 g

Sugar 3.9 g

Protein 1.8 g

Cholesterol 14 mg

Easy Lemon Chicken Soup

Difficulty Level: 2/5

Preparation Time: 10 minutes

Cooking Time: 10 minutes

Servings: 2

Ingredients:

1 1/2 lbs chicken breasts, boneless

3 cups chicken stock

1 tbsp fresh lemon juice

1/2 tsp garlic powder

1/2 onion, chopped

Pepper

Salt

Directions:

Add all ingredients except lemon juice into the inner pot of Pressure Pot and stir well.

Seal pot with lid and cook on high for 10 minutes.

Once done, allow to release pressure naturally. Remove lid.

Remove chicken from pot and shred using a fork. Return shredded chicken to the pot.

Stir in lemon juice and serve.

Nutrition: (Per serving)

Calories 676

Fat 26.2 g

Carbohydrates 4.4 g

Sugar 2.6 g

Protein 99.9 g

Cholesterol 303 mg

Basil Zucchini Soup

Difficulty Level: 2/5

Preparation Time: 10 minutes

Cooking Time: 15 minutes

Servings: 4

Ingredients:

2 zucchini, chopped

2 tbsp fresh basil, chopped

30 oz vegetable stock

1 tbsp garlic, minced

2 cups tomatoes, chopped

1 1/2 cup corn

1 onion, chopped

1 celery stalk, chopped

1 tbsp olive oil

Pepper

Salt

Directions:

Add oil into the inner pot of Pressure Pot and set the pot on sauté mode.

Add onion and garlic and sauté for 5 minutes.

Add remaining ingredients except for basil and stir well.

Seal pot with lid and cook on high for 10 minutes.

Once done, allow to release pressure naturally for 10 minutes then release remaining using quick release. Remove lid.

Stir in basil and serve.

Nutrition: (Per serving)

Calories 139

Fat 4.8 g

Carbohydrates 23 g

Sugar 8.7 g

Protein 5.2 g

Cholesterol 0 mg

Tomato Pepper Soup

Difficulty Level: 2/5

Preparation Time: 10 minutes

Cooking Time: 20 minutes

Servings: 4

Ingredients:

1 lb tomatoes, chopped

2 red bell peppers, chopped

1/2 tsp red pepper flakes

1/2 tbsp dried basil

1 tsp garlic powder

6 cups vegetable stock

2 celery stalk, chopped

3 tbsp tomato paste

1 onion, chopped

2 tbsp olive oil

Pepper

Salt

Directions:

Add oil into the inner pot of Pressure Pot and set the pot on sauté mode.

Add onion, red pepper flakes, basil, and garlic powder and sauté for 5 minutes.

Add remaining ingredients and stir well.

Seal pot with lid and cook on high for 15 minutes.

Once done, allow to release pressure naturally for 10 minutes then release remaining using quick release. Remove lid.

Blend soup using an immersion blender until smooth.

Serve and enjoy.

Nutrition: (Per serving)

Calories 134

Fat 7.7 g

Carbohydrates 16 g

Sugar 10 g

Protein 3.2 g

Cholesterol 0 mg

Sausage Potato Soup

Difficulty Level: 2/5

Preparation Time: 10 minutes

Cooking Time: 20 minutes

Serve: 6

Ingredients:

1 lb Italian sausage, crumbled

1 cup half and half

1 cup kale, chopped

6 cups chicken stock

1/2 tsp dried oregano

3 potatoes, peeled and diced

1 tsp garlic, minced

1 onion, chopped

1 tbsp olive oil

Pepper

Salt

Directions:

Add oil into the inner pot of Pressure Pot and set the pot on sauté mode.

Add sausage, garlic, and onion and sauté for 5 minutes.

Add the rest of the ingredients and stir well.

Seal pot with lid and cook on high for 15 minutes.

Once done, allow to release pressure naturally for 10 minutes then release remaining using quick release. Remove lid.

Stir and serve.

Nutrition: (Per serving)

Calories 426

Fat 29.1 g

Carbohydrates 22.3 g

Sugar 2.8 g

Protein 18.9 g

Cholesterol 78 mg

Roasted Tomatoes Soup

Difficulty Level: 2/5

Preparation Time: 10 minutes

Cooking Time: 5 minutes

Servings: 2

Ingredients:

14 oz can fire-roasted tomatoes

1 1/2 cups vegetable stock

1/4 cup zucchini, grated

1/2 tsp dried oregano

1/2 tsp dried basil

1/2 cup heavy cream

1/2 cup parmesan cheese, grated

1 cup cheddar cheese, grated

Pepper

Salt

Directions:

Add tomatoes, stock, zucchini, oregano, basil, pepper, and salt into the Pressure Pot and stir well.

Seal pot with lid and cook on high for 5 minutes.

Once done, release pressure using quick release. Remove lid.

Set pot on sauté mode. Add heavy cream, parmesan cheese, and cheddar cheese and stir well and cook until cheese is melted.

Serve and enjoy.

Nutrition: (Per serving)

Calories 460

Fat 34.8 g

Carbohydrates 13.5 g

Sugar 6 g

Protein 24.1 g

Cholesterol 117 mg

Basil Broccoli Soup

Difficulty Level: 2/5

Preparation Time: 10 minutes

Cooking Time: 15 minutes

Servings: 6

Ingredients:

1 lb broccoli florets

1 tbsp olive oil

1 tsp chili powder

1 tsp dried basil

6 cups vegetable stock

1 onion, chopped

2 leeks, chopped

Pepper

Salt

Directions:

Add oil into the inner pot of Pressure Pot and set the pot on sauté mode.

Add onion and leek and sauté for 5 minutes.

Add the rest of the ingredients and stir well.

Seal pot with lid and cook on high for 10 minutes.

Once done, allow to release pressure naturally for 10 minutes then release remaining using quick release. Remove lid.

Blend soup using an immersion blender until smooth.

Serve and enjoy.

Nutrition: (Per serving)

Calories 79

Fat 2.9 g

Carbohydrates 12.1 g

Sugar 4 g

Protein 3.2 g

Cholesterol 0 mg

www.ingramcontent.com/pod-product-compliance
Lightning Source LLC
Chambersburg PA
CBHW070734030426
42336CB00013B/1971